BETTER DAILY SLEEP HABITS

BETTER DAILY SLEEP HABITS

Simple Changes with Lifelong Impact

RENATA ALEXANDRE, PHD, APRN

ROCKRIDGE
PRESS

For general information on our other products and services or to obtain technical support, please contact our Customer Care Department within the United States at (866) 744-2665, or outside the United States at (510) 253-0500.

Rockridge Press publishes its books in a variety of electronic and print formats. Some content that appears in print may not be available in electronic books, and vice versa.

TRADEMARKS: Rockridge Press and the Rockridge Press logo are trademarks or registered trademarks of Callisto Media Inc. and/or its affiliates, in the United States and other countries, and may not be used without written permission. All other trademarks are the property of their respective owners. Rockridge Press is not associated with any product or vendor mentioned in this book.

Author photo courtesy of Ascension Health.

ISBN: Print 978-1-648-76977-1 I eBook 978-1-648-76978-8
R0

I dedicate this book to my family, for always being supportive of my professional endeavors. Especially my son, Brandon Bowers, who was helpful with the psychological aspects of this book, and my sister, Carol Deterding, who is always available to talk when I get stuck.

CONTENTS

INTRODUCTION

Getting a good night's sleep seems like it should be the most natural thing in the world, but for many of us, it isn't. According to the Cleveland Clinic, over 70 million Americans live with sleep disorders. If you're among that number and curious about lifestyle changes that can improve your sleep, you've come to the right place.

Not being able to get consistent, restful sleep can be incredibly frustrating. I know from experience. Prior to changing my sleep, the problem that impacted my sleep habits the most was anxiety. To address how anxiety was affecting my sleep, I learned several coping mechanisms and got help from a mentor who did a few sessions of cognitive behavioral therapy (CBT) with me. At first, it seemed like a long and arduous journey, and at times I questioned whether the benefits outweighed the hard work required to change my long-standing habits. But I'm glad I persisted, because the new habits I adopted help me to this day. For example, as I was writing this book, there were a couple of nights when I woke and had difficulty getting back to sleep. Now, when I relapse, I realize that I'm under stress, and I know how to get my sleep stabilized thanks to the coping mechanisms I learned all those years ago.

In addition to having personal experience with sleep struggles, I have worked as a certified nurse practitioner specializing in sleep medicine and the treatment of insomnia for 13 years, have a PhD in health and human performance, and have studied complementary and alternative medicine. The techniques you will learn in this book are those that I have found to be the most successful in my personal experience as well as in my clinical experience. The trick is to turn these techniques into habits so they become automatic.

In part 1, I'll give you some background about sleep and forming good habits. In part 2, I'll cover eight common issues that affect sleep, and for each one, I'll provide comprehensive guidance on how to develop positive sleep habits and break detrimental ones. Don't feel like you have to adopt every single strategy discussed in each chapter. Some will work better for you than others, because your situation is unique. The goal is to find a combination of techniques that are best for helping *you* successfully get to sleep and stay asleep. In addition, when you open your mind to the ideas set forth here, you may also find inspiration to come up with some of your own solutions.

I know that creating new habits and making lifestyle changes can be challenging, but the benefits to your health and well-being are well worth the effort. Remember, good habits are worth the energy and the time it takes to develop them, and small changes over time add up to remarkable results. Good luck on your journey to achieve consistent, restful sleep.

HABITS AND SLEEP

Consistent, restful sleep is one of the central pillars supporting a healthy life. Adequate rest for the body and mind increases mental clarity and processing ability, allows for the repair and rejuvenation of muscles and tissues, and improves the function of the body's systems.

Positive daily sleep habits provide a road map for the body to follow when it comes to getting to sleep and staying asleep. Once formed, these habits become automatic and lead to a lifetime of good sleep for most individuals.

In part 1, you'll learn how good habits and good sleep go hand in hand. I'll explain the purposes and benefits of sleep, the stages of sleep, and the impacts of sleep deprivation. I'll also discuss good and bad habits, how and why bad habits are formed, and the importance of adopting good habits and breaking bad ones.

CHAPTER 1

How to Have Better Sleep

In this chapter, you'll learn why sleep is necessary, starting with a definition of sleep and then moving on to how sleep affects the body, how the body facilitates sleep, and the different types of sleep. You'll also learn what disrupts or inhibits sleep, and the consequences of sleep deprivation. On the flip side, you'll learn how sleep improves learning and performance and how to establish sleep habits and good sleep hygiene.

Improve Sleep, Transform Your Life

Sleep is a restful state in which your awareness of and reactions to external stimuli are dramatically reduced. Your mind and body facilitate your ability to go to sleep and stay asleep. They do this by releasing hormones that promote sleep and by gradually cooling your body temperature as you move through the stages of sleep.

Sleep itself allows the mind to process emotions and consolidate memories. Additionally, it allows the body to repair cells, tissues, and muscles and to resupply resources that were depleted during wakefulness, such as hormones, neurotransmitters, and proteins. Sleep also enables the body to conserve energy in preparation for the day ahead.

There are two basic types of sleep and four sleep stages. The two types of sleep are REM (rapid eye movement) sleep and non-REM sleep. The four stages of sleep are: non-REM transition to sleep, non-REM light sleep, non-REM deep sleep, and REM sleep. During each stage, the body and mind focus on specific restorative tasks. During a typical night of good sleep, you will cycle through these stages four to five times.

During non-REM sleep, memories and experiences gained throughout the day are moved from short-term storage to a more permanent storage vault in the brain. During the non-REM deep sleep stage, memories are distilled and reflected upon.

Dreams are believed to occur during REM sleep. The brain wave activity of REM sleep is very similar to that of wakefulness. During this stage of sleep, the body is partially paralyzed: a protective mechanism that prevents you from acting out your dreams. Dreams are thought to foster emotional and mental health, in that dreaming about painful, difficult, or traumatic experiences can provide some guidance and resolution upon waking. Dreams are also thought to help you find creative ways to deal with a variety of daily concerns. Additionally, during REM sleep, experiences and memories from the past and present are synthesized to build a better and more accurate framework of the world we inhabit.

Despite what occurs in the mind and body to enable sleep, there are many things that can interfere with sleep. Some of the major causes of sleep challenges include stress, lifestyle choices, food, substances, medications, and supplements.

Stress: Stress impacts sleep by keeping your brain engaged in an issue that you often have no control over. Stressors can inhibit the ability to fall asleep and keep you from getting back to sleep if you wake during the night. Stressors are common in a well-lived life. Stress can be managed with daily habits that reduce the body's response to stress. You will learn more about these habits in chapter 9.

Lifestyle: Some lifestyle factors can be controlled more easily than others. One thing that you can control is your activity level. A life of activity and exercise enhances sleep by increasing the secretion of endorphins (a.k.a. "happy hormones"), keeping weight under control, reducing our risk for certain diseases, and reducing stress.

You'll find detailed advice on exercise habits in chapter 6. The time of day you work is something that's harder to control. But the good news is that sleep problems related to shift work can be managed with appropriate daily habits. I will discuss this more in chapters 4 and 5.

Food, Substances, Medications, and Supplements: Heavy foods such as pasta and potatoes, as well as sugar, caffeine, and alcohol, can interfere with sleep by having either a stimulating effect on the brain or increasing your body's core temperature, which must be cool to enhance sleep. Sleeping medications are generally best only for short-term sleep needs because in the long term, they can worsen sleep. Antihistamines, melatonin, and valerian can each help in different ways in the short term but typically cause an unpleasant hangover effect.

The lack of adequate restful sleep can reduce physical performance, weaken the immune system, increase cognitive decline, and worsen cardiovascular disease, mood disorders, and weight gain. It is also implicated in increasing substance abuse. Studies show that the cognitive impairment in those with sleep deprivation is equivalent to the impairment seen with blood alcohol levels over the legal limit. In addition, sleepiness impacts the mood negatively, makes learning difficult, affects memory, and reduces the ability to obtain good grades.

Healthy, Restful Sleep Matters

The renewal of the body and brain that results from restful sleep has additional life-enhancing effects, from improved learning performance to greater alertness while you're awake.

Sleep prior to learning helps refresh your ability to make new memories and thereby learn new things. For instance, studies show that napping between learning new tasks replenishes the brain and makes learning more successful and efficient. Sleeping well the night after learning is also beneficial because it consolidates and helps you retain what you've learned. If you want to remember something, read it over prior to going to bed at night. Your memory of the subject matter will be enhanced when you awaken the next morning.

On the other hand, sleep can also help you forget things you don't want to remember. A 2019 study published in *Cellular Neuroscience* had subjects focus on words to remember and words to forget. Those who slept after studying the list of words were better able to remember the words they were supposed to remember and to forget the words they were supposed to forget.

Sleep enhances the performance of many other tasks, as well. A 2009 study of musicians found that adequate sleep prior to a performance increased the accuracy of their playing. This was also true of typists who were studied after sleep. Sleep helps athletes recover more quickly from post-performance inflammation and muscle breakdown, and plays a critical role in recovery after a stroke, as new neural networks are organized and recover their function.

Finally, and perhaps most important, sleep is important for daytime wakefulness, alertness, and safety. In a world where sleep deprivation has become a way of life, the National Highway Traffic Safety Administration reported that an estimated 91,000 car crashes in 2017 were the result of "drowsy driving." In the wake of statistics such as this, new rules have arisen to ensure that commercial drivers (as well as airline pilots) are well-rested before they navigate their equipment.

Develop Your Sleep Habits

Often, when people first take up an activity, their concentration effort is high, most likely because they are attempting to solve a problem they have not previously encountered. Once they determine how to best deal with the issue at hand, their response gradually becomes more and more automatic. Soon, they begin to do the activity without even thinking about it.

Now, think about this process in the context of your sleep. Imagine trying to determine what can make you sleep better or consulting an expert about how you can sleep better. There are several sleep activities with which you can begin. For example, let's say you're a nighttime clock watcher. You've been told to stop this behavior by a sleep expert, so you take the clock out of the bedroom. Once you are accustomed to the absence of the clock, you don't think about its absence, especially when you are sleeping better. Having no clock by your bed has become a way of life—or a habit.

Sleep hygiene is a collective name for the many habits that enhance sleep, including regulation of the sleep period; restricting time in bed for sleep, intimacy, and sickness; and adjusting daily activities to enhance sleep. If you make sleep hygiene practices into habits, sleep improves. As with most habits, the more you perform them, the better you get at them, and the better you get at these habits, the better you sleep.

The more associations you can make with your bed and sleep, the easier sleep becomes. Sometimes that means planning your entire day so that you can enhance your ability to get to sleep and stay asleep. The more your brain thinks about sleep when you see your bed, the easier it will be to find rest.

This means that habits that are negatively impacting your sleep goals will need to be changed. One such habit that is prevalent in today's world is playing games or checking social media on our phones while lying in bed or upon waking in the night. There are several reasons to avoid this negative habit, which I will address later; however, the individuals I have treated who have successfully stopped this habit were amazed at how it changed their sleep for the better.

Similarly, a good sleep habit that I often see in those who are accustomed to routine is a stable wake time. They have made a stable wake time a priority and stick with it. These individuals typically have very little difficulty with their sleep.

In the following chapters, you will learn more about how to form good habits and break bad habits related to bedtime routines, including those related to establishing a stable sleep schedule, stress management, regular exercise, dietary habits, and changing your sleep environment to optimize sleep.

KEY TAKEAWAYS

- Sleeping well renews the body and mind. Allowing for this renewal not only enhances your physical and mental state, but it also improves your ability to learn and perform, and keeps you alert and attentive while you're awake.
- Developing good sleep habits can enhance sleep. When you practice good habits, they become automatic, and sleep improves.
- Changing your sleep habits is possible. You can learn good sleep habits and unlearn bad sleep habits. You'll learn more about how to accomplish both of these things in the chapters to come.

CHAPTER 2

What Are Habits, and Why Do They Matter?

In this chapter, you'll learn more about habits and how they are established. You'll also learn about what is happening in the brain when habits are formed and when they're changed. Finally, you'll see how small daily changes can make a big difference for your sleep, especially when bad habits become good habits.

Habits 101

The brain is constantly making predictions based on your experiences and your environment. These predictions guide your behavior. For instance, if you predict a positive outcome, you are more likely to engage in behaviors that could potentially lead to that outcome. In addition, if your prediction matches your desired outcomes, you will likely continue those behaviors.

When you experience an outcome that aligns with your desires more than once, your brain intrinsically analyzes all the data that is coming in during those experiences and develops expectations about future events and automatic behaviors if the experience is repeated often enough. For example, if you notice that every day the sun comes up in the east, your brain makes the prediction that tomorrow when the sun comes up, it will appear on the eastern horizon. In your personal and emotional life, you make similar predictions. If every time your mother sang a song, you felt a sense of joy as a child, likely when someone important to you sings a song today, you continue to feel that joy. The sense of joy has become an automated response to hearing singing. The reason this occurs is because it has become an automatic response. Your orientation to a joyful response matches your sensory input.

Habits work in much the same way. When a specific stimulus has occurred repeatedly, your brain and body respond in a similar way every time they encounter that stimulus. This is especially true for routine behaviors, such as developing habits to optimize sleep. At first a conscious effort is required, but with repetition, the response becomes automatic. When it is habitual, we no longer need to think about it; we simply act. When the activity becomes unconscious, it is a habit.

Habits can be broken down into several parts. In the next section, I'll describe each of these parts and explain their role in what is called "the habit loop."

The Habit Loop

The body is always searching for ways to reduce energy output and increase efficiency. Activities we perform regularly, or habits, are one avenue to achieving the body's goals. The habit loop is a process the brain learns to help the body conserve energy by consistently responding to certain stimuli with the same behaviors.

There are three parts to the habit loop. First, there's a cue, or a trigger. The response to the cue is called the routine, which is a behavior carried out following the cue. Finally, there's a reward, which is what you get out of the situation. If the brain likes the reward, it will continue to respond to the cue in the same way in the future.

We are often engaged in habit loops without knowing it. When I was young, I learned how to use many different tools and machines to accomplish various tasks. I would consistently leave the tools out after I used them. When I needed to use those same tools again, I sometimes had difficulty remembering where I was when I last used them, and they would be "lost" for a short time. This caused me a great deal of frustration. So, I began to put my tools in a designated place after each use (something that my parents had tried to teach me but I had ignored).

The cue became a lost tool, and eventually simply use of a tool. The new routine became putting the tool away after each use. And the reward was having my tools available to me whenever I needed them.

What's Happening in the Brain

In the brain, habits are formed by repetition. The cue causes neurons in the brain to fire. When you choose a specific path, or routine, repeatedly, the same neurons are activated and create a track in the brain. Over time, this track gets deeper and deeper, and at some point, you no longer need to choose the path—the neurons automatically send you down the same path that was previously chosen.

Habits, therefore, are a process. Initially, you need to think through multiple options and consciously choose the path you want to take. Over time, after you have chosen the same path (or routine) repeatedly, your brain's response to the cue becomes instinctive—you no longer need to think about it. This habit will continue indefinitely as long as the reward has value to you.

Sometimes habits begin unintentionally. In other words, you are faced with a problem that requires a solution. You discover a way to solve the problem, and each time the problem recurs, you solve it in the same way. But it's very likely that you never consciously consider that you're forming a habit or whether the routine has a positive or negative impact on your life. This is true especially of day-to-day habits.

What About Bad Habits?

Bad habits are routines that interfere with how we live our lives. Bad habits are easy to develop because they offer immediate gratification as a reward. Once a negative habit loop is established, its corresponding track in the brain will not go away. When new, healthier habits are formed, completely new tracks are formed, but the old tracks remain. The more you have performed a behavior, the deeper the track is, and the harder it is to avoid it when you're stressed. That's why emotional strain often triggers a return to bad habits.

Many bad habits develop in response to environmental factors that trigger changes in behavior. These behavioral changes may or may not be beneficial in the long-term. For instance, when the COVID-19 pandemic began, many people started working from home. Because most no longer needed to commute, some may have filled this extra time by watching TV or sleeping. These more sedentary habits, while they may offer immediate gratification, may also have resulted in weight gain or insomnia or both.

Bad Habit Loop

The habit loop is similar for good and bad habits. The difference is that a good habit may or may not involve a craving. Bad habits almost always involve a craving followed by an emotional response to the craving. The bad habit loop, therefore, has a cue, followed by a craving and its emotional response, then a routine, and lastly a reward. When emotions become involved, we do not necessarily form habits that will benefit us, because the craving is difficult to resist, and the reward being sought often involves immediate gratification.

In many cases, bad habits occur as a response to a particular stressor and don't involve forethought about the long-term outcomes; therefore, the routine ends up only superficially solving the problem, compounding the problem, or complicating your lifestyle to a degree that will require later remediation. For example, Julie adopted Ginny, a poodle. In the first weeks after bringing the puppy home, Julie put Ginny in bed with her to stop the dog's nighttime crying. It worked well until the puppy grew into a 70-pound dog and Julie got married and had a husband, Ron, to share her bed. Julie's cue had been the crying at night, her desire was to get sleep, and her frustration caused her to adopt a solution without a lot of forethought. Julie could have made this a good habit loop by putting Ginny into a kennel and using simple training methods to help Ginny get comfortable being on her own at night. Though this routine requires delayed gratification, it is a better long-term solution that won't cause Julie or Ginny stress in the future.

Breaking Bad Habits

Developing a bad habit is easy. Breaking a bad habit is more difficult. It often takes a change of environment to break the habit, because bad habits are frequently a response to a cue that evokes a specific desire. To break a bad habit, you need to change a part of the habit loop.

First, think through the habit loop (cue, craving, routine, and reward) for the habit you want to change. Once you have considered these elements, you can begin to change the habit by blocking something in either the routine or the surrounding environment. In the case of Julie and Ginny, when Ron moved in with Julie, Ginny needed to get out of the bed. Ginny responded once again by crying at night. Knowing they would move homes soon, they began to help Ginny get into a new routine of energetic activities so that she was tired prior to bedtime. When they made the move into their new house, their new routines helped Ginny acclimate to her surroundings and to the new sleeping situation.

A change in routine and environment is often necessary to break a bad habit. Sometimes a fundamental change in how you view the habit and its effect on your life may be required.

Small Changes, Big Results

Changing your habits can be hard, but remember that as you repeat a new, more positive routine, it will become easier and more automatic, with the cue or the craving putting you on the path to a healthy and satisfying reward. Over time, the benefits of good habits are compounded.

In his book *Atomic Habits*, James Clear explains that if you get 1 percent better at a habit every day, over the course of a year, you will be 37 times better at the habit you have developed. Imagine the improvement after five or ten years of performing the same daily habit. Take reading, for example. If you started reading as a young child and developed a habit to read every day, you are probably still reading as an adult. Over time, not only did reading became easier, but it likely improved your vocabulary and contributed to your understanding of the world, yourself, and other people. When you apply this concept to your career, it may seem to others as if your successes appeared overnight. If you look back on your daily work habits, however, you will likely recognize how good habits have increasingly bolstered your career and helped you become successful over time.

There are several methods you can use to change your lifestyle and adopt new habits. One of the simplest ways is to maintain the cue and the reward but change the routine. This is especially helpful if your routine is what is causing problems. A workout routine of jogging is no longer helpful when arthritis in your knees is causing you significant pain. The cue can still be putting on your running shoes, and the reward will still be the good feeling the endorphins give you after working out, but you may need to bicycle rather than run.

Another option is to use a technique called "habit stacking," which is when you pair an enjoyable habit with one that you have difficulty performing. Perhaps before you shower, you clean the sink or toilet. Or before you sit down to watch your favorite show, you wash the dishes.

A new environment can also be a catalyst for habit change. For example, if you're sensitive to light, having blackout curtains on your bedroom windows or opening the curtains every morning and closing them at night may improve your ability to stay asleep.

I'll discuss all of these, and additional techniques, more specifically in the coming chapters.

KEY TAKEAWAYS

- Habits are created to solve problems efficiently. The brain wants to do everything with as little energy as possible, and habits facilitate this type of efficiency.
- Bad habits compound over time and can be a source of problems.
- The benefits of good habits also compound over time. The longer you have a good habit, the more benefit you receive from it.
- It is possible to change habits. Using several different behavioral methods, you can develop new tracks, or habit loops, in the brain that offer positive rewards.

PART 2

BUILDING HEALTHY SLEEP HABITS

Sleep is influenced by many factors. In a sense, your day consists of a series of routines that predict your ability to sleep at night. In this section, I'll discuss several sets of habits that you can develop to optimize your ability to sleep. Following a sleep schedule is the most important step you can take to improve your ability to get to sleep and stay asleep. I'll begin there and follow it with habits that will improve the association between your bed and your sleep, such as developing a sleep routine and establishing a healthy sleep environment. Then, I'll move toward other activities that influence your sleep such as stress reduction, exercise and timing of exercise, food and the timing of our meals, exposure to screens, and time outdoors. In the final chapter, I'll explain how practicing mindfulness can improve your sleep.

CHAPTER 3

Following a Sleep Schedule

I n this chapter, you'll learn how to develop and keep regular sleep times as a way to help establish healthy sleep. Your brain and body seek out routine, so when you establish a schedule and engage in consistent behaviors related to sleep, it becomes much easier to get to sleep and stay asleep. Your brain is also constantly making associations between the world around you and your behaviors. When you look at your bed, you want the association to be with sleep. A sleep schedule can help make this happen.

Why a Sleep
Schedule Matters

A consistent sleep schedule creates a positive habit loop by providing cues for the time to prepare for sleep, the time to go to bed, the time to wake up, and the time to get out of bed and start the day. A sleep schedule improves sleep quality and efficiency because it reinforces positive associations and teaches your brain and body to take the path, or develop the routine, that is rewarded by healthy, restorative sleep.

Everyone has a sleep need, which is the number of hours that our bodies have the capability of filling with sleep every night. If your sleep need is 7 hours but you spend 10 hours in bed each night, your sleep will most likely be fragmented, and you will be as tired as if you got 5 hours of sleep. A feeling of sleepiness can make you think you didn't rest for long enough, but it's more often the case that you didn't get the consolidated sleep your body needs.

Most people tend to do better when they are able to satisfy their sleep need all at once and during night-time hours. The circadian day then begins in the morning when you wake up. This means that the part of your sleep schedule that you should most closely maintain is your morning wake-up time.

Between approximately 11:00 a.m. and 3:00 p.m., your body may crave sleep. If siestas, or daytime naps, are not part of the culture you've grown up in since childhood, giving in to napping during this period can interfere with your ability to get good, consolidated sleep at night. This is because it decreases your drive for sleep. So, in general, it is not a good idea to nap during the day. Instead, plan to be active during this period.

Building Healthier Habits

There are a few simple ideas to remember when you are building healthier habits. Healthy habits are easier to create and maintain if they are easy to do and fit well into your current routines, you enjoy doing them, and they make sense to you.

Whether you go to bed early or you're a night owl, the five key habits in this chapter will bring consistency to your sleep schedule so you can easily fall asleep at bedtime, stay asleep during the night, and wake up ready for your day. They will help you become more aware of your sleep needs and help you create positive associations between your bed and sleep. Finally, these habits will provide solutions for when something disrupts your sleep schedule, from late-night social activities to waking in the middle of the night.

Because your sleep schedule is the cornerstone of good sleep hygiene, establish the habits in this chapter before moving on to the habits in other chapters. I strongly recommend spending time on all of the habits in this chapter because they will have the greatest impact on the quality of your sleep.

Establish a Stable Wake Time

If you change nothing else but this habit, your sleep will improve. You could choose to work on stabilizing your bedtime or wake time (and you may eventually do both), but starting with establishing a stable wake time works best for most people because it mirrors the natural world.

An army veteran told me that he used to sleep very well due to the regimented beginning of his day at 5:00 a.m. When he got out of the service, he began sleeping longer on weekends, spending more time in bed than he could fill with sleep. This behavior caused him to have difficulty getting to sleep on weekdays and resulted in difficulty getting out of bed. Eventually he started sleeping nearly entire weekends thinking he needed more sleep. That is when he came to me. We changed one habit: He was to get out of bed at the same time every day. He started sleeping better and feeling better approximately two weeks after his wake schedule stabilized.

The best wake time to choose is the earliest time you need to wake up during the week. This is your cue. Then, set an alarm to get out of bed at your wake time. This is your routine. Then, choose an enjoyable activity—many people work out, meditate, or read. This is your reward. Once out of bed, proceed to your activity and have fun beginning the day.

Establish a Stable Bedtime

A stable bedtime is especially important during the work-week, so you can get the rest you need to competently perform your duties and obligations. But if you struggle to maintain a regular bedtime, you might be surprised to learn that your weekend habits may be the source of your problem. Getting to bed at a stable time facilitates getting up at the same time every morning, so changing your schedule on the weekend is not a good idea. If you do have a late night, make a point of getting out of bed at your normal wake time so that you are ready to resume your bedtime schedule on Sunday night.

Once a month Janice enjoyed a Saturday night out with "the girls." They enjoyed their social activities often until the early morning hours. Janice always had difficult Mondays and Tuesdays because she slept longer on Sunday morning and had difficulty getting to sleep on Sunday night. After some thought, she decided to set her alarm on Sunday morning for the same time as she set it on weekdays, even after her nights out. She no longer had difficulty getting up early during the week.

Choose your bedtime. This is your cue. If falling asleep prior to bedtime has become a habit, set an alarm on your phone for your bedtime, and when it sounds, go to bed. If you are not sleepy, refer to the next habit. Your routine is simple: crawl into bed. Your reward is being able to wake up at your scheduled wake time feeling refreshed.

Go to Bed When You're Sleepy

This habit strengthens the association your brain makes between your bed and sleep. If you go to bed and ruminate about the day or become anxious about what may happen tomorrow, your brain will associate worry and anxiety with sleep. Spending time tossing and turning prior to going to sleep reduces the quality of your sleep, and you are more likely to awaken feeling much less refreshed. If you go to bed sleepy, you are more likely to get to sleep quickly and establish positive connections in the brain between your bed and sleep.

Janet was a psychologist who worked with college students. A student, Karen, was a freshman in college and was having difficulty getting to sleep at night. Karen shared with Janet that she was going to bed at 9:00 p.m., despite not getting sleepy until midnight. Janet simply suggested she go to bed at midnight. Not only did Karen get to sleep more quickly, but she was much more alert during the day.

For about a week, spend some time while you are waiting for sleep to arrive to write in a journal. As part of your journal entries, keep track of when you begin to feel sleepy. The feeling of sleepiness is your cue. The routine is to go to bed when you are sleepy, but not before. Your reward is being sleepy enough to fall asleep easily. After a week, review your journal entries and use the time that you tend to feel sleepy as a guide for the next habit.

Control Light Exposure to Reinforce Your Sleep Schedule

Dimming the lights in your home in the evening reduces stimulation to the brain and helps produce melatonin, a substance that helps our brains to sleep. Conversely, getting light into the eyes in the morning stimulates the brain and helps it wake up. Controlling light exposure is particularly helpful for night owls and people who work swing shifts or night shifts.

Dillon worked from 7:00 p.m. to 7:00 a.m. He would fall into bed and have difficulty getting to sleep, even when he was exhausted. He was not having difficulty staying asleep during the day because he was by nature a night owl. He just had difficulty getting to sleep. He came to see me, and I suggested that he wear sunglasses on his way home from work to prevent the sunlight from stimulating his brain. I also suggested that he get blackout curtains to avoid light during his sleep time and to avoid flip-flopping his schedule on days off. When Dillon returned to my office, he was sleeping and feeling better.

As part of your bedtime routine (see chapter 4), dim the lights an hour before bedtime (Dillon wore sunglasses). A book light is usually fine because it does not shine in your eyes. At your established bedtime, darken the room completely. This is your cue to go to sleep. In the morning, open the curtains or turn on the light. This is your cue to wake up and start your day. Your reward is getting to sleep more easily and being more fully awake and alert in the morning.

Get Out of Bed

There may be times when you wake in the night and have difficulty returning to sleep. If you lie in bed and allow your mind to race and your emotions to be triggered, you will find it very hard to return to sleep. To interrupt anxious nighttime thoughts, get out of bed and take worries to another room.

John woke every morning at approximately 3:00 a.m. to use the bathroom. Often, he had no difficulty returning to sleep, but occasionally, he would still be awake when his alarm sounded. He would begin the day upset because of lack of sleep, and this mood generally lasted all day.

One night, he simply got out of bed and meditated. When he went back to bed, he got to sleep quickly, and despite his interrupted night, he was able to function well the following day. He now practices this habit consistently.

Waking in the night is your cue. This is your routine: Pay attention to your body's cues. If you begin to become emotionally frustrated because you cannot get to sleep, get out of bed. Do something that will help you fall back to sleep, such as reading (with a book light), listening to calming music, or practicing mindfulness (page 137). Do NOT turn on the TV, use your phone or computer, or undertake an activity that requires anything more than dim light or you will further awaken your brain. Returning to sleep is your reward.

Breaking Bad Habits

There are two habits that can interfere with your ability to successfully follow a sleep schedule: napping and lingering in bed. These habits can negatively influence your ability to get to sleep at your established bedtime, stay asleep throughout the night, and consequently maintain a stable wake-up time. They also can interfere with or disrupt the positive habits and associations that you will be creating related to your sleep schedule.

Although overcoming bad habits can be challenging, it's not impossible. It's easier to break bad habits if you make them difficult to act on or if they don't fit into your current schedule.

Both of these strategies will work well for breaking these particular habits.

Napping

Napping is a habit that typically forms in the absence of a regular sleep schedule or when your personal sleep need is not being met. Individuals who reduce their nighttime sleep during the workweek just to get everything done tend to nap after work or on weekends to "catch up." This is inefficient. If you get the right amount of sleep every night, you have no need to catch up, and every day is a high-functioning day on the sleep spectrum. Unless you are ill (or have specific needs due to a sleep condition like narcolepsy or being a long sleeper), avoiding naps is an important sleep management tool.

Bill is 72 years old. He came to me with difficulty getting to sleep at night. His sleep schedule had not changed in 50 years, but after he retired, he added a regular one- to two-hour nap after lunch into his daily schedule. Approximately two weeks after he did this, he began to have difficulty getting to sleep. He really enjoyed his nap and did not want to give it up, but when he did, he began to sleep like he did when he was working. Bill wanted to get as much sleep as he could to improve his daily functioning. Unfortunately, it did not improve his day, but made it worse. When it comes to sleep, more is not necessarily better.

Lingering in Bed

Lingering in bed is something that many people like to do on weekends or days off. Lingering in bed while on the phone or watching TV allows the brain to create associations between the bed and these activities rather than with sleep.

The more often one of these alternate activities is repeated, the more ingrained the habit loop will become in the brain. This is how problems begin.

I am a night owl with a four-and-a-half to five-hour sleep need. My bad habit is lingering in bed. I don't play on my phone or watch TV—I doze. When I first developed my sleep schedule, this was my most difficult habit to break. I scheduled activities I enjoyed for the early morning hours, so that I would get out of bed. It took about a year to fully break my old habit, but now I wake every morning at 4:30 a.m. and get up to do some sort of exercise. Not only does it solve the lingering issue, but it also gives me energy all day long.

Tracking Your Progress

This tracker can help you monitor your progress as you make changes in your sleep schedule. The first four healthy habits on this list are those that you want to maintain long-term. Though getting out of bed is a good habit, you want to see the frequency decrease over time as your ability to sleep through the night improves. Also, track your bad habits, the frequency of which should also decrease over time. In addition, there are several blank rows for you to fill in with other good or bad habits you want to work on. The more you are able to see that you are consistent with the changes you have made, the more likely you will be able to maintain them. Ultimately, that is the goal.

HABIT	M	T	W	TH	F	SAT	S

KEY TAKEAWAYS

- The most important part of your sleep schedule is your wake time. If you can make your wake time stable every day of the week, you will sleep much better.
- Track when you get sleepy at night and use this to establish a stable bedtime. If you happen to stay out late one night, set your alarm and wake up at your established wake time to maintain your sleep schedule.
- Give your mind and body sleep and waking cues by controlling your exposure to light. As you prepare for bed, dim the lights. Just before you go to sleep, darken the room. When you wake up, let the light in!

- Getting good quality sleep hinges on the positive associations your brain makes between your bed and sleep. When the brain makes associations between the bed and other activities, your sleep can be negatively impacted.
- Tracking your progress is one of the best ways to ensure your success. It becomes harder and harder to break the chain of success as you add more and more days of positive practice. And the more days of success you add, the more habitual your behavior becomes.

CHAPTER 4

Establishing a Bedtime Routine

O ptimal sleep occurs when your sleep habits are stable and consistent. In developing a bedtime routine, you will be building powerful associations with sleep. The habits in this chapter will especially help you with getting to sleep and may even help you stay asleep through the night. Repetition of the same or similar routine every night prior to going to bed is key.

Why a Bedtime Routine Matters

Establishing a bedtime routine provides a series of signals to the brain that you're about to go to sleep. These habits become the cues to slow down and relax. After a busy, stressful day, it is often difficult for the brain to decompress. A bedtime routine provides the time and space for the brain to unwind and release any tension that has built up over the day.

Taking the time to allow your brain to relax is similar to allowing your muscles to relax after vigorous exercise. If you have a cool-down period at the end of your exercise routine, you reduce your risk of injury and strain. The same is true of your brain. It requires time to wind down, and a bedtime routine provides that.

Often, we fill our pre-sleep routine with activity, but it is more conducive to develop a routine that is less active. This time and space allows our brain to enjoy something pleasurable prior to sleep. The more often you do the same activity prior to bedtime, the stronger the association becomes and the easier it is for sleep to arrive.

Some quiet pursuits that can help your brain release the stresses of the day include reading, meditating, praying, coloring, knitting, and doing crosswords. If you choose to read, this is the time to pick up something that is interesting but easy to put down at any time, not a page-turner. Do not read or do puzzle games on a screen; when preparing for bed, use paper versions.

When bedtime arrives, you should be able to fall asleep easily once you have established the routine. It does take some time for the brain to begin making the association, but usually within two weeks you will see some positive changes.

Building Healthier Habits

In this chapter, you will learn habit stacking, where the first habit will be a cue for all the other habits. In other words, you will begin with a cue that leads to a routine, which becomes the cue for your next routine, and so on.

One of the easiest ways to begin a new habit is to tie it to another habit that you already perform. If you tell yourself that you will brush your teeth after you put on your pajamas, you tie these habits together. The more you repeat these habits together, the more seamless they become. Over time, they become one combined action.

Ordering your habits in the same way every night is an important part of the process. Any small change that is made in a routine upsets the procedure and has the potential to halt the entire series of habits. At first, you may need to write yourself a list so you do all these routines in the same order. You will no longer need a list once the series of routines becomes a habit.

A bedtime routine complements your sleep schedule by preparing your brain and your body for sleep. When you take time to calm your mind and body, you send a message to the brain that you are winding down for the day, allowing it to gently pass to the next phase of your day.

Turn Electronics Off

In the previous chapter, you learned about controlling light exposure before bed to reinforce your sleep schedule. At the point in your sleep schedule when you dim the lights, you'll also want to turn off all electronic devices. This should occur approximately one hour prior to bedtime. Electronic devices include the television, computers, cell phones, and tablets (including those used to read e-books).

Many people are sensitive to light, and that includes the light generated from electronic devices. The screens on electronic devices are backed by blue light, which suppresses melatonin production.

Cindy grew up afraid of the dark. When she was young, she always had a night-light in her room. Over time, she got into the habit of reading in her bed prior to sleep. Often, the bedside light stayed on all night. When she turned 45, she began to have difficulty sleeping and could not understand why. A sleep clinician told her to turn her light off and resume using a night-light. One month after beginning this new habit, she was getting to sleep and staying asleep much better.

Set an alarm for one hour prior to bedtime. The alarm is your cue. Your routine is to turn off all electronic devices and dim the lights. Your reward is being able to fall sleep and stay asleep easily.

Get Active Tasks Done

Any activity that requires energy or movement should be done before you settle into a more relaxing pursuit. These activities include brushing teeth, combing hair, and showering or bathing. Getting your active tasks done early reduces stimulation of the brain and maintains calm as you invite sleep. Think of these tasks as the effort you expend prior to the cooldown in your exercise routine. Often, the most vigorous part of your workout comes at the end just before you cool down, recover your breath, and let your muscles slowly release. Similarly, these tasks are the final effort in your day before you allow your brain to rest.

Jack learned in the military that the more active he was prior to bedtime, the harder it was for him to get to sleep. He began to sit down and read prior to bedtime. Then, he would get up and shower before going to bed. Unfortunately, he would again start actively thinking about things during or after his shower. Jack decided to reverse his routine by showering first and then sitting down to read. He was amazed that such a simple change could help so much; he's had no problem with getting to sleep since he changed his routine.

Stack this habit with the previous habit: turning off your electronics. Your cue is turning off your electronics and dimming the lights. The routine that should immediately follow is getting all your active tasks done. Your reward is having a relaxed mind and body when you get into bed.

Prepare the Bed Area and Put Your Pajamas On

This habit will follow, or get stacked with, the previous habit. After you have completed your active tasks, turn down your comforter and put on your pajamas. Also, check the bedside area to ensure that you have every-thing you need for the night—for example, earplugs or a night mask. Make sure anything you need is lying close by so you don't have to get up to hunt for it after you are already settled in bed.

Jane is a swimmer. Her husband snores, and she uses her swimming earplugs in bed to drown out the noise. She forgets to put her earplugs beside the bed when she gets home from swimming and often needs to retrieve them when she is ready to get into bed. When she forgets her earplugs, she gets frustrated with herself. She often needs to read again to calm down enough to get to sleep. She began to retrieve her earplugs when she turned off her electronics, which has eliminated the frustration and difficulty getting to sleep.

The cue for this habit is the completion of your active tasks. Your routine is to move directly to the bed and turn back the covers, put on your pajamas, and make sure that everything you need for sleep is close by. Your reward is the ability to get to sleep easily without interruptions.

Engage in a Relaxing Activity

Engaging in a calming activity works best when the specific activity is something that you do only prior to bedtime. If you like to read, perhaps this is when you read magazines or a specific genre of books. Being consistent about the type of activity creates a strong and very spe-cific association between relaxation and sleep, cuing the body and mind to slow down. Allow plenty of time for this activity to invite relaxation, typically 30 to 45 minutes.

Martin was diagnosed with coronary artery disease and had his first stent placed after a bout of chest pain. He was surprised by the illness and the diagnosis, and worried about his mortality. The evenings were especially worrisome because he had more downtime. He would worry all evening and have difficulty getting to sleep. In the cardiac rehabilitation program, he learned that coloring relaxed him. He could fall asleep after he colored, an unexpected bonus for him. He made coloring part of his bedtime relaxation routine and rarely had difficulty getting to sleep after that.

The cue for this habit is the completion of preparing your bed area and putting on your pajamas. Your routine is then to engage in your chosen relaxing activity. Your reward is the ability to be sleepy at bedtime and getting to sleep quickly.

Relax Your Mind and Welcome Sleep

When your mind and body are relaxed, you can close your eyes and let consciousness recede into the background. This allows sleep to arrive much more easily. Going to bed before you are in a relaxed state leaves the door to active thinking ajar in the mind and can sabotage your efforts to relax and prepare for sleep.

Martin colored every night prior to bedtime because he found that coloring relaxed him. The only time that Martin had difficulty going to sleep was when he did not wait until he was completely relaxed and sleepy. He habitually went to bed at a very specific bedtime, whether he was fully relaxed and sleepy or not, because the time of day was a strong cue for him. When he learned to recognize when he was fully relaxed and sleepy, his exact bedtime fluctuated slightly, but he rarely had difficulty getting to sleep.

The cue for this habit is engaging in a relaxing activity. Your routine is to assess your relaxation and sleepiness at your scheduled bedtime. If you are not fully relaxed and sleepy, continue your relaxing activity or change to journaling as suggested in chapter 3 (page 25). Your reward is having a calm and relaxed mind at bedtime so you can get to sleep faster.

Breaking Bad Habits

It can be difficult to begin a sleep routine if you already have a set of behaviors that are working against your ability to get to sleep. This is especially true if you have become attached to these behaviors. Bad habits, as stated previously, often offer immediate gratification, and that's why it can be hard to break them.

When bad habits begin to affect your health or, in this case, your ability to sleep, the motivation to make changes becomes more serious. Sometimes you simply need to remove distractions from easy reach or to a different room. But sometimes you may need to ask for help from others or ask them to respect certain boundaries. These are not unreasonable requests.

The two most common habits that cause sleep disruption are using a cell phone when waking during the night and being too responsive to requests from others. The mobile phone, even when placed in night mode, has enough light to stimulate the brain to wakefulness. Being responsive to others is a virtue most of the time, but if it interferes with your sleep or your ability to get to sleep, it is detrimental.

Using Electronics in Bed

Playing games or checking social media in the middle of the night is not conducive to good sleep. Though many people have no difficulty getting to sleep again after light stimulation, the quality of sleep suffers and, over time, sleep deprivation occurs. When you turn off your electronics (including your cell phone), leave them at the opposite end of your house or apartment from where you sleep. If you need to have your phone close in the event of an emergency, put it on the opposite side of the room so you need to get out of bed to retrieve it.

Cindy woke at least twice every night to check social media. She enjoyed the contact with her friends and her family and could be caught laughing in the night at some of the things she read. Over time, even when she did not have her phone with her, she woke at the same times every night to check her phone. Eventually she started noticing daytime consequences: She began arriving late to work and got sleepy at her desk. She was at the point of losing her job when she arrived in my office. When she stopped checking social media in the night, it took only a month before she was once again sleeping through the night and back to her previous energy level.

Being Overly Responsive to Others

Everyone has different sleep requirements that need to be protected, so placing boundaries on the time you will be available to others is extremely important. Although there are times and situations when this can be challenging—especially for caregivers, such as parents of young children or those caring for a sick or elderly relative—making a concerted effort to protect your sleep means you'll be alert and responsive when you need to be. Moreover, during times of stress, it is especially important to protect your sleep, because sleep deprivation can compound anxiety and may diminish your capacity to deal with complex situations.

It is important to communicate with your family and friends about your sleep needs to ensure that they respect your boundaries. It also helps to agree on a definition of what is considered an emergency.

Fred's wife died when his youngest child was 5 years old. He raised his children on his own and was very responsive to their needs growing up. His youngest child was 23 when I met Fred, and his adult children were still interrupting him at all hours of the day and night with things that he considered frivolous. He tried talking with each of them but had little success. Fred finally had a family meeting with all three of his children and their families. He informed them that he would be available only from 8:00 a.m. to 10:00 p.m. If they had an emergency, they were to call Fred's neighbor who had agreed to notify Fred during the noncommunication hours. It took some time, but Fred no longer is being called throughout the night.

Tracking Your Progress

The sleep habits in this chapter can be stacked on one another. If you like, you can view it as one routine with five steps. By tracking your good and bad bedtime habits you create a record of your progress. The tracker holds you accountable and encourages you so you're more likely to be consistent. Each time you engage with one of your new habits, you are one step closer to it becoming an automatic behavior, and each time you look at the tracker, you are reminded of your goals. Use the spaces at the end of the tracker to add any good or bad bedtime habits you want to work on.

HABIT	M	T	W	TH	F	SAT	S

KEY TAKEAWAYS

- Stacking habits is a good way to develop any sort of routine. By performing related tasks together, you build one big habit loop. Once that habit loop is established, the only cue you'll need is the first cue.

- The association you make between sleep and your bed can be strengthened by performing the habits in this chapter in consecutive order. This pre-sleep routine (all five habits) will help you relax from your day so you can fall asleep quickly, but it may also help you sleep through the night.

- Turning off electronic devices of all kinds at least an hour before bed and keeping them far from your bed during the night is a critical habit to develop in order for your bedtime routine to be successful.

- Getting active tasks done before you prepare your bed area, put your pajamas on, and engage in a relaxing activity will help ensure that your mind doesn't revert to an active state and interfere with your ability to get to sleep.

- When you are engaged in your relaxing activity, make sure you give yourself enough time to let your mind fully relax. If you are not fully relaxed and sleepy, it will be more challenging to fall asleep.

CHAPTER 5

Changing Your Sleep Environment

Your sleep environment, including the temperature of the room, the noise level, and the comfort of your bed and bedding, also plays an important role in your ability to get a good night's sleep. When all these items are considered, sleep can be effortless. The ideal conditions for sleep are not the same for every person, and challenges can arise if you sleep in the same bed as someone who has different preferences than yours. In that case, you may need to compromise. The goal is to make the environment comfortable for everyone.

Why Your Sleep Environment Matters

Not everyone has problems with their environment, so the habits in this section can be developed individually or stacked as necessary to address any of the particular challenges you might be experiencing. There are sound physiologic reasons why some items in your bedroom environment can have a negative impact on your sleep, while other things are simply a matter of comfort. There are four basic elements that you should consider when you are thinking about your sleep environment: noise, temperature, light, and comfort.

Noise can help with sleep or hurt it. The types of noise that can help with sleep are white noise and pink noise. White noise is a form of sound that has an equal intensity across all tones audible by the human ear and is helpful to drown out other ambient noises. Pink noise is similar, with the exception that deeper tones are louder than higher pitched tones, making it a softer sound for the human ear.

The comfort of your bed and your bedding is an obvious facilitator of sleep, yet it always surprises me how many people sleep with pillows that do not provide a comfortable night's rest or keep a mattress far longer than it is capable of being supportive or soothing. There are many products on the market that can make your sleep more comfortable. Start with affordable basics, like comfortable sheets and good pillows. If you need a new mattress, which is more of an investment, be sure to do your research, go to the store and test different styles if you can, and look into payment plans and return policies.

Building Healthier Habits

You may or may not be experiencing problems with your sleep environment. If you are not, it's still worthwhile to pay attention to it and know what makes you most comfortable. Sleep changes with age, primarily due to health issues such as pain and the introduction of medications, so having an awareness about the conditions that best facilitate sleep for you is important. This awareness can help you adapt your environment as necessary to maintain your ability to sleep when such issues arise.

The habits in this chapter can be stacked on one another or stacked as needed with the bedtime routine habits in chapter 4. Some habits naturally complement one another. For example, engaging in a relaxing activity (page 40) allows the body's core to cool down and prepare for sleep. If you set your thermostat to a comfortably cool temperature at the same time that you dim the lights and turn off your electronics, it will further encourage your body to gravitate toward sleep. Also getting pets settled in their night routines as part of getting active tasks done (page 58) is a natural habit pairing.

Because your ideal sleep environment is unique to you, there may be additional habits not mentioned here that will increase your comfort. If that's the case, use what you've learned about habit loops and habit stacking to identify and develop any additional habits that will improve your sleep environment and track them in the habit tracker at the end of this chapter.

Find a Comfortable Bedroom Temperature

Too much heat in the bedroom can cause sweating, and too little heat can cause shivering. Finding the right temperature can be challenging, so you may have to experiment a little bit. Try setting the thermostat at slightly different temperatures for a couple of nights. If you do not have a thermostat, you can use a fan or open a window to cool the room. Using light, breathable sheets or heavy blankets are other options when it's difficult to precisely control the temperature in the room.

Jerry and Lisa were both having difficulty with the bedroom temperature at night. Jerry was sweating in the night when the thermostat was set to Lisa's preferred room temperature, and Lisa would wake shivering when it was set to Jerry's preferred temperature. The setting on the thermostat was a common source of arguments. Because it is easier to add blankets and wear warmer pajamas, they decided to get some supplies. Now they are both comfortable with the room temperature set at Jerry's preference. Lisa is now equipped with fleece-lined pajamas and a couple of extra blankets. Both are now sleeping much better.

Remembering to set the thermostat can be a challenge if it is not already part of your evening habits. To begin this habit, set an alarm for an hour before your established bedtime—this is your cue, and it can also work as your cue to beginning your bedtime routine (see chapter 4). The routine: Turn down the thermostat to the desired temperature. The reward is being comfortable when you fall asleep and not waking up in the night due to being too hot or too cold.

Create a Dark Sleep Environment

Ambient light shining into your bedroom can keep you from getting to sleep and staying asleep. It can also wake you in the morning. A 2018 study in the *Journal of Psychiatric Research* shows that even small amounts of light in the bedroom can interfere with sleep and recommends the use of an eye mask. Even the lights on electronics showing they have power can pose a problem. As a one-time routine, check the bedroom for any light. Lights on devices can easily be covered by black tape, and blackout curtains are an option if your current curtains don't do an effective job of keeping your room dark.

Jesse left his bedroom television on all night from the time he was approximately 15 years old. He liked the light in the event he woke in the night. At age 42 he arrived in my office because he was having difficulty getting back to sleep after waking in the night. He did not think it was the light of the television. After dealing with other sleep hygiene issues, he still was not able to stay asleep. He took the TV out of his bedroom. Within three weeks, he was having very few issues with staying asleep.

The first habit in your bedtime routine is a great cue for the routine of closing your curtains at night. Or you can stack it with setting the thermostat (page 56), getting active tasks done (page 42), or preparing your bed area and putting your pajamas on (page 43). In any case, prior to putting on pajamas, close the curtains. You will be rewarded with a dark room that facilitates falling to sleep easily and getting a restorative night's sleep.

Block or Drown Out Noise

Some individuals become acclimated to ambient noise. Others find it interferes with sleep. Earplugs work well to block noise, if you can sleep with them. White noise or pink noise can drown out environmental noise. Binaural beats, in which tones register differently in each of your ears, are known to decrease anxiety and invite sleep. Songs with binaural beats can be found on YouTube and other music apps (if you do use a phone app, make sure to place the phone across the room). Other forms of white noise include the whir of a fan or the sounds of a humidifier or CPAP machine.

Gail lived in an apartment that was above a heavily traveled street. She was very sensitive to noise but was unable to tolerate earplugs. I saw her when I was home on vacation and introduced her to white noise. A few months later she called me to let me know that she had found a white noise app that provided the perfect sound to drown out the environmental noise.

This habit can also be linked to your bedtime routine. When you begin your bedtime routine, simply use one of your existing habits as a cue and stack turning on the white noise or putting earplugs on the bedside table with getting active tasks done (page 42) or preparing your bed area and putting on your pajamas (page 43). Your reward is the absence of jarring noise as you drift off to sleep.

Train Your Pets

If you have difficulty getting to sleep or staying asleep, having a pet in the bed can be a hassle. For some, having a pet in bed with them is a comfort. Unfortunately, as we age, small disruptions in sleep can cause bigger problems, so it's generally a good idea to teach your pets their own separate sleep routines when they first come home with you. This is the easiest time to train your pet. Trying to train them after they've already been in your bed is not impossible, but it is more challenging.

Grayson adopted a puppy. He had a dog previously that woke him up constantly in the night. When he adopted his new puppy, he decided he would begin a new nighttime routine for the dog. Prior to his own bedtime routine, he began a nighttime routine for the puppy: play for a bit, go outside, and go into the kennel. This routine began the first night the puppy was in Grayson's apartment, and after a few nights, the puppy anticipated the routine and did not cry.

This habit can be stacked on other habits during your bedtime routine, with the cue being whatever task you choose to pair it with. The key is to do it before you engage in your relaxing activity. The routine: Perform your pet's routine, then put them into a kennel or a closed room away from the bedroom. The reward: no nighttime or early morning disruptions.

Select Comfortable Furniture and Bedding

Comfortable surroundings facilitate better and more sound sleep. You learn over time which supplies you need to sleep well. Some like a lot of pillows and others prefer none. The important thing is knowing what is right for you, so you are comfortable enough to fall asleep easily.

Basic items include a comfortable mattress, pillows, sheets, and blankets. Other items that may support your sleep include different types or sizes of pillows, wedges, weighted blankets, and comforters of different weights and warmth ratings. When these accessories appropriately support your head and body, sleep comes easily. When you wake with aches in your back, neck, and hips, it may be time to get new equipment.

Ella loved her mattress. After she purchased it, she began to sleep like a dream. Now, however, she is waking in the night with her hips aching and is not feeling as refreshed when she wakes in the morning. Her friend, Sue, got a new mattress and was bragging about how well she was sleeping. After she did some research, Ella was stunned to realize that her mattress was 12 years old. She replaced her mattress and is now sleeping much better.

Stack this habit with preparing your bed area and putting on your pajamas (page 43). Your cue is when you turn down the covers on your bed. Your routine is to arrange your accessories in a way that makes you most comfortable. Your reward is that your bed is always a haven for sleep so you can get to sleep quickly and wake up well-rested and pain-free.

Breaking Bad Habits

Sometimes bad habits occur due to a lack of boundaries. Setting boundaries related to sleep expectations will help you better manage your sleep routines and gives those you live with some guidance about those expectations. Boundaries will be different for each person. You might consider some of the following questions when you set your own boundaries:

→ How hard is it for you to get to sleep and stay asleep?
→ If you wake in the night, do you have difficulty getting back to sleep?
→ Are you pleasant when you wake up in the morning?
→ Are you a night owl or a morning lark?

Substituting a good behavior for a bad behavior can be an effective way to halt bad habits, which is how we will manage the two common bad habits that I see frequently in my work related to sleep habits.

Allowing Pets to Disturb Your Sleep

Dogs and cats can both become destructive if you simply close the bedroom door to them. Anticipate their frustration and provide another option for them. One of these is finding something to entertain your pet through the night. A toy or treats that they are allowed only at night can help your pet adjust. Leaving the window curtains open with a light on outside allows pets to entertain themselves by watching what is happening in the lighted area outside the window.

Another option for both cats and dogs is training them to sleep in a bed of their own or in a kennel. A kennel is probably the most difficult option if a pet has been on your bed since they were very young. Offering treats when the pet goes in its kennel or its own bed can help them acclimate to this setup.

Jeremiah adopted a rescue dog that was accustomed to sleeping in bed with his previous owner. Jeremiah purchased his pet a comfortable bed and placed it at the bedside. Every time the dog laid on its bed, he got a treat and plenty of attention. It did not take long for the dog to stay on the floor and in its bed.

Watching the Clock

Watching the clock is a common bad habit. When you watch the clock due to anxiety, you tend to calculate the amount of time you have left to sleep and place pressure on yourself to get to sleep again. If sleep does not return, frustration occurs. Once emotions are involved, it is very difficult to get back to sleep at all. The remedy is simple: Turn your clock away from you so that you cannot see it in the night. In addition, refrain from looking at any other timepiece if you wake in the night.

Jordan came to see me because he was unable to stay asleep at night. He always woke at approximately 3:00 a.m. He needed to get out of bed by 5:00 a.m. to get to work on time. Jordan was a night owl, so getting to sleep was difficult, and he had slept through his alarms enough times that he became anxious that he would not be able to wake with the alarm. In his anxiety, he awoke two hours before his alarm sounded, began calculating how much time he had left to sleep, and often had difficulty returning to sleep. At first, he resisted turning his clock away from him, but when he did, he found that after a few nights, he no longer woke early to check the time and was able to sleep through the night.

Tracking Your Progress

Many sleep environment habits can be added to your bedtime routine. Tracking these behaviors will help you remember to perform them and will also give you a record of your successes. As you find it easier to get to sleep and stay asleep, and your habits become more automatic, you may not need to track your activity as closely. But come back to the tracker during times of stress, when the possibility of reverting to bad habits is greater. Tracking your habits during these times will help you get through the harder times and ensure that you are getting the sleep you need to competently deal with life's complexities.

HABIT	M	T	W	TH	F	SAT	S

KEY TAKEAWAYS

- Your sleep environment can easily facilitate or inhibit sleep. Optimizing your bedroom to maximize your comfort and minimize disruptions while you are going to sleep and during the night will result in improved sleep quality.
- Most problems that arise related to your sleep environment involve noise, temperature, and light.
- Although having pets in bed is often desired by pet owners, and may be a comfort to some, pets are also a source of sleep disruption. Train your pet to sleep on their own or provide special toys or treats to ensure that both you and your pet get adequate sleep.
- Assessing the comfort of your sleep environment and developing habits that ensure your comfort will help facilitate sleep. It is simply more difficult to fall asleep and stay asleep if you are uncomfortable.

CHAPTER 6

Getting Physical

R outine exercise enhances sleep. In this chapter, you'll learn why exercise is so important to getting quality sleep and how to develop an exercise routine that will benefit your ability to sleep. The many advantages of an exercise routine include reduced risk of diseases, endorphin release, effect on body temperature, and reduction of stress—all of which positively influence sleep quality. I'll discuss this in more detail in the pages that follow.

Why Physical Activity Matters

Staying active is important for good health in general, and it has specific benefits for sleep. Engaging in physical activity outdoors is especially helpful for sleep, because it adds a circadian rhythm component that influences your ability to get to sleep and stay asleep. (I'll explain more about how getting outdoors benefits sleep in chapter 10.)

On the most basic level, the expenditure of physical and mental energy that occurs during exercise is tiring, so it makes getting to sleep easier. This energy release also fosters your ability to stay asleep as the body uses this time to repair itself from being active.

Exercise, however, has additional benefits related to sleep. It raises your core body temperature and keeps it elevated for a long period of time. This helps you stay awake and energized because it elevates your metabolism. When your metabolic rate goes up, you are better able to stay awake and engaged in your daily activities. When you are less sedentary throughout the day (and avoid napping), you are more ready for bedtime when it arrives. In addition, as your core body temperature cools, you become sleepy and find it easier to get to sleep.

Physical activity, especially strenuous physical activity, also reduces stress. The reduction of stress and anxiety makes getting to sleep and staying asleep easier. Exercise also increases the production of neurotransmitters in the brain called endorphins. Endorphins naturally augment your overall feeling of well-being. Endorphins may also help you stay awake during the day, which increases your drive for sleep at night, as well as the likelihood that you will enjoy a sound and restorative sleep.

Building Healthier Habits

Not everyone likes exercise, and many of us have tried to begin an exercise program and found it daunting. The habits in this chapter were chosen with this in mind. The goal here is to develop habits that will support you as you begin an exercise routine and will make it easier to get the exercise you need to improve your sleep.

When you're developing any new habit or routine, but especially an exercise routine, it's crucial that your goals are achievable. Make sure that both the type of exercise and the time investment are reasonable and practical for you. Simply put, if your routine is not doable, you will not do it.

Another way to keep up with your exercise routine is to develop habits that involve accountability. You will have days when your motivation flags, and you can't rely on willpower alone to keep yourself going. With established positive accountability habits, your response to these challenges will be automatic: when you experience the cue, your accountability routine will kick in and keep you on track.

Finally, exercise shouldn't be boring. Some people love doing the same exercise every day because it's predictable, but most people need some variety. Varying the type of exercise you do during the week not only will help you stay healthy and fit but will also fend off boredom and prevent lapses in your exercise routine that could negatively affect your sleep.

Increase Repetitions Gradually

When starting a new exercise program, people often think that there's a specific number of repetitions they "should" do for it to qualify as exercise. This idea is counterproductive, and it could lead to a discouraging level of soreness, pain, or even injury. Pain and injury can also disrupt your sleep. Plus, you'll need to cut back or even stop exercising in order to recover, which may also affect your ability to fall asleep and stay asleep.

Start simple by doing one repetition of your chosen exercise. Do one sit-up (or any other exercise) today. Then increase the repetitions gradually by adding one sit-up every day until you reach your daily goal. If you are sedentary, one sit-up may actually help your sleep because you'll be more active than you were yesterday. This method is an easy way to make your new exercise routine doable.

Gerald wanted to restart exercising and was having difficulty getting started. When asked how much he could easily do, he said three burpees. He does burpees three days per week. He began adding one repetition every day. By the end of the month, he was doing 15 burpees. He also noticed that the physical exercise was helping his sleep.

First determine when you would like to exercise. Perhaps the ideal time for you is before breakfast. Your cue is the time of day (before breakfast). Begin with one repetition (or how many you can easily do without overexerting yourself) of the exercise you want to begin with. Each day you perform that exercise, add one repetition. Soon you will be dividing your repetitions into sets (instead of 10 repetitions per set, do two sets of five). This is your routine. Continue to do what you can comfortably and avoid overdoing it. You want to continue this habit, so staying comfortably within your limits is very important. Your reward is sounder, deeper sleep.

Increase Time Gradually

Some exercises do not have repetitions per se. With these you can gradually increase the amount of time you spend doing the activity. Walking is a good example. You generally do not need to count your steps, though you can if you want to with the use of a fitness watch. Walking, jogging, biking, and swimming can be timed. If you start with a five-minute walk and add one minute every time you walk, it won't take long before you are walking for 30 minutes.

June was a swimmer, but she was unable to engage in that activity for approximately six months for health reasons. She wanted to begin swimming again, but her first time back in the pool was discouraging. She began by swimming only one minute. She added one minute of time each time she swam after that first time back in the pool. In one month, she was swimming consistently for 15 minutes. She also found that she was sleeping much better on the nights after she swam.

As with the exercise repetition habit, tie this habit to a time of day or a day of the week. This is your cue. Begin your exercise of choice by engaging in it for as long as you can comfortably. Add one minute each time you repeat the exercise. Continue to add one minute to your routine until you reach your goal. This is your routine. You will likely find that as you increase your time exercising, you will also increase your ease at getting to sleep and staying asleep. This is your reward.

Use a Habit Tracker

Habit tracking is a good way to monitor your progress and encourage yourself to be consistent. It's common for people not to recognize how well they are doing at developing new habits until they record their accomplishments on paper and have something physical to look at. When you begin feeling encouraged by the boxes checked off and discouraged when you miss one, you are well on your way to making your new exercise a habit.

It can also be helpful to use your tracker to record the quality of your sleep. You will likely find that you sleep better when you exercise consistently.

Henry made a New Year's resolution to begin an exercise routine. He did not keep track of the times he exercised or of the exercises he was doing. Initially he noticed that his sleep significantly improved when he started; however, he would exercise five days a week one week, and then skip an entire week because his body was too sore to exercise. His sleep was equally erratic and seemed to correspond to his exercise schedule. A trainer at his gym suggested he track his exercise. He began to exercise more consistently, avoid soreness from overdoing it, and began to sleep much better on a consistent basis.

This habit can be stacked on your exercise routine. Your cue is exercising. Your tracker will show on paper how successful you are at completing your goals and provide encouragement to continue. Your routine is documenting your exercise on your tracker. Your reward is the satisfaction of getting regular exercise and better sleep.

Work Out with a Buddy

When you work out with others, you are accountable to them and more likely to continue your exercise routine. Here are some suggestions:

→ Find someone at the gym you attend and work out with them on a specific day and time regularly.
→ Join exercise classes in which you exercise with a group.
→ On specific days, walk with neighbors or friends.

Don't forget that your workout buddy can be your pet! Walking your dog is a great way to get regular exercise, or volunteer to walk a neighbor or friend's dog. Elderly neighbors with pets may welcome having someone walk their pet on a regular basis.

Jane loved to exercise by doing aerobic dance. She often exercised at home using a TV program for dance as her guide. She found that she too easily avoided her exercise routine if a problem arose, and she became frustrated because she was starting to gain weight. With weight gain, Jane started to have difficulty staying asleep at night. An aerobic dance class opened at her gym and she joined. She started making friends in the class, enjoys the banter that goes along with the exercise, and now never misses a class. And as a bonus, she is now sleeping much better as well.

First decide what exercises you would like to do. This is your cue. Find an exercise partner for each form of exercise, to help you stay accountable to your exercise program. Exchange phone numbers so that you'll get a call if you miss your class or your exercise date with your partner. This is your routine. Once you are exercising regularly, you will find your sleep patterns changing for the better. This is your reward.

Add Variety and Consider Timing

Once you get your exercise routine established, you will likely want to add some variety to prevent boredom and the overuse of particular muscle groups. Again, start simple and work your way up. Add one or two exercises to the one you started with, or walk one day and start doing sit-ups (or the exercise of your choice) the next day. As you continue to become more advanced, you may consider doing a series of exercises that primarily work on your legs one day and your upper body another day, then do aerobic exercise on another day. Anytime you add an exercise to your routine, or choose a more vigorous exercise, start with a low number of repetitions (or amount of time), and slowly increase to reduce soreness and potential injury. In addition, varying what you do keeps you from getting sore and keeps the entire body exercised.

Exercising in the morning is also optimal. Exercise boosts your metabolic rate. This causes a greater expenditure of energy throughout the day, which in turn helps you sleep better at night. A 2018 article in *Everyday Health* suggests that when you exercise in the morning, you may sleep better, but picking the right time and the appropriate exercise for you is what's most important. When you sleep better, you have more energy to exercise, and the cycle repeats itself.

Dean was a night owl, and exercised after work at approximately 5:00 p.m. He was specifically working on upper body strength. He found that he was getting too sore to exercise every day, so he began to skip days. Soon he was not exercising at all. He visited a trainer at his gym who suggested a variety of exercises. Dean was no longer getting sore because each muscle group had a day or two to rest before he exercised again. This allowed him to change to a morning exercise schedule that fostered better rest at night.

Think about a variety of exercises you would like to do. This is your cue. Plan a short time every day to do your timing or your repetitions, preferably in the morning to get the best results in your sleep. Choose an exercise buddy for each exercise. This is your routine. Soon you will meet your exercise goals. Your reward is deeper, more restful sleep.

Breaking Bad Habits

Some people do not enjoy exercise, and others may enjoy the benefits of exercise but struggle with motivation. A common challenge related to these blocks is putting off exercise or making excuses. One way to address these challenges is to pair exercise with an enjoyable activity. For example, listening to music, a podcast, or an audio book while you walk. Or making a regular date to walk and talk with a friend. Pairing exercise with something you look forward to creates a powerful positive association in your mind that can help you maintain a more consistent exercise schedule. Mindfulness is another excellent way to address these problems (more on this in chapter 11).

When you're starting a new exercise program, it can be easy to fall into bad habits simply due to lack of experience. Your enthusiasm to achieve your desired results may cause you to overdo it to the point of exhausting a particular muscle group or suddenly finding yourself bored and unmotivated. Doing too much, too soon will quickly disrupt or derail your exercise routine. Therefore, it's important to find creative ways to maintain your interest and manage your output. It can be as simple as changing your walking route or checking websites like bodybuilding.com for new ways to strengthen particular muscle groups. You could also expand your list of exercise buddies.

The bottom line is that disruptions in your exercise routine can interfere with your ability to get to sleep and stay asleep. If you do find yourself falling into negative habit loops, take a moment to reassess, revisit the healthy habits in this chapter, and consult the advice that follows.

Procrastinating

Procrastination is detrimental to any type of activity, exercise included. It is easy to make excuses and start avoiding something that you do not particularly enjoy, and the more you allow yourself to avoid something, the easier it is to let it slide and forget about it. Stopping an exercise routine also halts the benefits that you obtain from the activity. Sleep will suffer if you put off your exercise routine.

Thankfully, there are some good ways to avoid procrastination. Having an exercise partner who will keep you accountable is often helpful. If you aren't friends already, you will likely develop friendships with your exercise partners, and it's hard to let friends down. Another solution is to join an exercise class that performs the exercise you're interested in trying or improving. For cyclists, joining a spin class will help you stay on track—and you may even develop friendships in your classes that will help keep you accountable.

Harry loved playing video games, which was his favorite activity before he went to work in the morning. He was gaining weight though, because he was spending so much time sitting. He also noticed that he was not sleeping as well. He needed to exercise. He joined the gym with a friend and they began working out together. Though many mornings Harry would have preferred to play video games, he did not want to disappoint his friend, Jim, by not showing up. He was able to lose weight as well, which was a bonus for him. With weight loss and the success of his exercise routine, Harry also had no difficulty with his sleep.

Overdoing It

If you already exercise or are excited about your new exercise routine, it's likely that you are consistently challenging yourself to do more. This can be good; however, it is possible to push yourself beyond your abilities, which often results in injuries or strains. If you do injure yourself, you will typically need to reduce or refrain from exercise for a period of time.

One way to avoid this is to keep an exercise journal. If you track how much weight you lift and how many repetitions you do rather than pushing your body until it can no longer lift, you can improve safely. Because your primary goal is to improve the quality of your sleep, there's no reason to overdo it. Injury and strain will only exacerbate your sleep problems.

Another way to avoid overdoing it is to enlist the help of an exercise buddy. Have someone who also exercises keep you accountable to a reasonable increase in your performance. If you do not have an exercise buddy, you can often ask questions of trainers or get involved in an online chat with trainers who can answer your questions.

Justin worked out regularly. He decided to enter a weightlifting competition. He had one year to get into shape. In the first weeks, he kept injuring his right arm. He awakened frequently in the night because of discomfort, fragmenting his sleep. As a result, he also noticed that he was sleepier. He enlisted the help of a trainer to find that he was simply increasing his weight too fast and needed to tweak his technique slightly. He was able to slow down and be in shape in time for the competition. He also found that he slept much better, which allowed his muscles to recover from his workout routine.

Tracking Your Progress

Keeping both a calendar of your activities and a log on distance, time, repetitions, and sets in your chosen activities is extremely helpful. A physical record of your progress will help encourage you and also prevent you from overdoing it. Although this habit tracker is a good start, I recommend also keeping a separate exercise journal where you can keep a more specific record of your activities.

HABIT	M	T	W	TH	F	SAT	S

KEY TAKEAWAYS

- Exercise helps you sleep by expending pent-up energy in the body. The type of exercise is immaterial to remaining active.
- Exercise can increase your energy during the day. With increased energy, you are often able to remain more active during the day, which makes you more tired at night, thereby ready for sleep at bedtime.
- When beginning an exercise routine, start simple and gradually build up repetitions or time.
- Boredom or overexertion can derail your exercise routine and consequently interfere with your sleep. Make sure to vary your activities and use a habit tracker, or check in with a trainer or exercise buddy to monitor exertion levels.
- Pick an exercise time that works best for you, but remember that the earlier in the day you exercise, the more energy you expend, and the easier it is to get to sleep and stay asleep at night.

CHAPTER 7

Eating Wisely

The timing of meals and the foods that you eat have a significant effect on your sleep. For instance, the timing of breakfast can impact how quickly you wake in the morning, and the timing of your evening meal can affect your ability to get to sleep and the overall quality of your sleep. The timing and composition of your meals can also make you sleepy or stimulate you at inopportune times. In this chapter, you'll learn how to adapt your eating habits so you can sleep better.

Why Eating Wisely Matters

When it comes to food, there are three basic things that affect sleep: alcohol, caffeine, and carbohydrates. Carbohydrates are further broken down into simple sugars and complex sugars. Each of these substances uniquely interfere with or enhance sleep. Problems arise when we misunderstand how these substances affect our sleep and we experience their effects at times when they are least welcome.

Although it's common for people to use alcohol to get to sleep at night, it's not a good idea. Alcohol is a depressant that enters the bloodstream very quickly, which is why it causes sleepiness. Unfortunately, it also leaves the bloodstream very rapidly after it's metabolized, which can disrupt deeper stages of sleep by causing brain stimulation. Even if this brain stimulation does not result in waking to full consciousness, sleep is still compromised and will be less refreshing.

Caffeine stays in the system for 10 to 12 hours. It typically does not prevent the ability to go to sleep, but it keeps you in the shallower stages of sleep for longer periods of time, thereby disturbing sleep quality.

A carbohydrate meal that contains simple sugars (sugar, corn syrup, lactose, and fructose) will provide energy for a short period of time; however, these sugars are digested rapidly. When digestion is complete, blood sugar levels crash, resulting in sleepiness. When this is coupled with the sleep dip that naturally occurs between

11:00 a.m. and 3:00 p.m., we are tempted to nap, which interferes with nighttime sleep quality.

Eating too close to bedtime warms the body core through the digestive process. Eating a meal high in complex sugars (pasta, vegetables, rice, and quinoa) in the evening will also interfere with sleep because of the length of time digestion requires. It is best to eat a light meal in the evening to ensure rapid digestion and enhance sleep.

Building Healthier Habits

Planning ahead for meals is similar to planning ahead for sleep. When you develop good eating habits, it will lead to improvements in your entire circadian day. Once established, eating habits are strong habits that tend to set the tone of our days. Just as exercise habits and sleep go hand in hand, so too do eating habits and sleep.

Eating wisely in this context means that the timing and the content of your meals supports wakefulness in the morning and afternoon, the ability to fall asleep easily at night, and the ability to satisfy your sleep need with the necessary amount of non-REM deep sleep and REM sleep. This means that eating habits should neither make you sleepy during the day, nor should they stimulate your brain at night. Furthermore, you will sleep much better if the digestion process from your last meal is completed before you begin your bedtime routine. This will allow the body to cool properly, which allows for better sleep.

Eat Breakfast

Eating breakfast every morning gives your body the fuel to accomplish the goals you have set for the day. Breakfast increases your metabolic rate early in the day to give you more energy to be active. The more active you are during the day, the easier it is to sleep at night. Breakfast does not need to be large. Establishing this habit is easy if you prepare your breakfast the night before so it's ready to go when you wake up.

Terri had difficulty waking up in the morning. She did not eat breakfast. She was told by her doctor that she needed to begin eating breakfast. This was a challenge for her because she really did not get hungry until later in the day. She decided she would have an apple every day for breakfast. After she cleaned her dinner dishes, she set the table for breakfast. On her placemat she placed an apple, a paring knife, a dish, and salt. She found it easy to begin the habit of eating breakfast daily, which resulted in being less sleepy in the morning and having more energy to get her day started.

After cleaning the kitchen table of dinner dishes, set your table for breakfast. Your cue is cleaning the dinner dishes. Your routine is getting your breakfast prepared as much as you can safely. Your reward is having your breakfast waiting for you when you get up in the morning, making it easy to sit down and eat.

Eat a Low-Carbohydrate Lunch

Eating a low carbohydrate lunch will help you avoid napping during the sleep dip during the late morning and the early afternoon. When you avoid napping, you improve your nighttime sleep by strengthening your drive for sleep. You can stack this habit with preparing breakfast.

Jeremy went to his car on his lunch break every day at work to eat his lunch and take a nap. He was having a sandwich, chips, and a soda each day for lunch. He didn't like taking a nap, but he couldn't make it through the day without one. He talked to his father, who'd had the same problem when he was younger, about it. His father suggested eating a different type of meal composed of protein and fresh vegetables and avoiding chips, breads, and sodas. When Jeremy changed his diet, he found that he no longer needed the lunchtime nap.

After you fix your breakfast for the following day, pack your lunch. Your cue is breakfast preparations. Your routine is packing the fruits, vegetables, and proteins you have chosen for your lunches and avoiding any sugary foods or drinks. Your reward is having the energy to get through the sleep dip.

Avoid Caffeine Within Eight Hours of Bedtime

Caffeine can keep you from sinking into the deeper stages of sleep by stimulating your brain. Because it's the deeper stages of sleep that satisfy your sleep need, getting into those stages improves the quality of your sleep.

Planning your meals helps you avoid caffeine too late in the day. When you drink caffeine too close to bedtime, you may find that you cannot get to sleep, which can cause frustration. When our emotions become involved, it can be doubly difficult to get to sleep. The best way to avoid this scenario is to avoid caffeine within eight hours of bedtime.

Gregory had difficulty getting deep sleep. He was an athlete and worked out daily in the evening, leaving the gym at 5:30 p.m. He drank caffeinated beverages and carbohydrates to aid in muscle healing. After visiting with me, Gregory changed his workout time to the early morning. Within two weeks he felt as though he was getting better quality sleep and felt more refreshed when he woke in the morning because he was no longer drinking caffeine in the afternoon.

First plan your meals for either a full week or one day at a time. If you plan for a full week, your cue is making your grocery list. If you plan for one day, your cue is time—when you clear your dinner dishes. Plan your meals for the following day, including beverages. Calculate eight hours prior to bedtime and plan no caffeine after that time. Your reward is more satisfying sleep.

Avoid Alcohol Within Four Hours of Bedtime

It may be tempting to use alcohol to help you get to sleep because it initially makes you very sleepy, but this is bad idea for two reasons. First of all, relying on alcohol for this purpose is discouraged because of the risk of abuse and addiction. Furthermore, alcohol will bump you out of the deeper stages of sleep if you ingest it too close to bedtime. Generally, it takes the liver four hours to metabolize alcohol, so if you have a drink at 9 p.m., you will likely experience a sleep disruption around 1 a.m.

Penelope had difficulty getting to sleep at night. She came to me to get a sleep aid. In our discussion, she offered to try alcohol. I suggested that she avoid alcohol because she would likely need more and more over time to maintain sleep. I suggested she begin a bedtime routine. She immediately started and did well. She was thankful she did not begin using alcohol for sleep and does not drink alcohol within four hours of bedtime.

Your cue is planning your meals. When you plan meals, also plan for beverages, including alcohol. Calculate four hours prior to bedtime and avoid alcohol after that time. You may sometimes feel compelled to have an alcoholic beverage at social events out of politeness or obligation. If this occurs, a nonalcoholic choice is a good option. Your reward is getting a satisfying night of rest.

Eat Dinner Four to Five Hours Before Bedtime

Timing your dinner four to five hours prior to bedtime provides time for digestion and allows the body core time to cool.

What you have for dinner can also affect your sleep. There is currently some investigation into the relationship between the foods we eat, the health of our digestive system, and sleep. Though science has not yet caught up with what we see clinically, we can still do a few things to improve the quality of our sleep. According to a 2020 article in *Everyday Health*, some studies suggest that taking probiotics may improve gut health and sleep. Eating a dinner meal low in processed foods and sugars also helps. My patients have improved the quality of their meals and often sleep much more soundly without making any other changes to their sleep habits.

Millicent had sleep apnea. She was also diagnosed with diabetes. She went on a diabetic diet and began to eat healthier meals. She had always eaten dinner about three hours prior to going to bed. She was unhappy with her sleep quality, even with CPAP, so she also began to have her evening meal earlier. Not only did her diet have a positive effect on her diabetes symptoms, but she found that she also slept better.

Calculate the time four to five hours prior to bedtime. The time of day will be your cue. Your routine is making a healthy evening meal. Enjoy it. Your reward is getting better quality sleep.

Breaking Bad Habits

There are many bad habits that we very innocently get ourselves into when it comes to eating and sleep. Not maintaining a regular eating schedule is one of those. If your meals are not timed thoughtfully, they will negatively impact your sleep. In today's world, it's easy to eat spontaneously, which often causes trouble. Keeping to a schedule lets the body know what to expect so it can function more efficiently.

Another bad habit related to eating and sleep is choosing too many unhealthy foods and not enough healthy ones. Sometimes food fads and food marketing mislead us. For instance, when I was a child, we were told that oleo (margarine) was a much healthier choice than butter. Now we know that trans fats, which are high in oleo, are worse for us than butter. Other bad habits related to food choices include a tendency to reach for carbohydrate-heavy comfort foods or highly processed foods when we're stressed–or even sometimes when we're feeling happy and celebratory.

In order to select foods that will keep us healthy and help us sleep, it's important to be able to discern between fads and fact, and to keep up on changes in food science. It's also important to put thought and care into what we eat, because our bodies are a holistic mechanism, so the choices we make about one thing, like eating, naturally affect many other bodily systems and processes.

Making Poor Food Choices

Making poor food choices has many implications because social activities revolve around eating. Processed foods offer quick energy, have more calories, and have less nutritional content than foods made from fresh meat, fruits, and vegetables. Fast foods are processed foods that have the same effect on the body as ready-made meals found in the freezer section at the grocery store. Many of our favorite foods also have a high sugar content.

Substituting sweet treats with fresh fruits and vege-tables and making our own meals at home are effective ways to break this habit. Just as you gradually increased repetitions in your exercise routine (page 70), gradually increase the amount of fresh food you use in your meals. Assess how much fresh food you're currently eating (if that is none, then start with one meal) then make one more meal during the week using fresh food. Gradually increase this by one meal each week. Before you know it, you will be enjoying meals made from fresh food regularly.

Adeline did not like to cook. She purchased many microwave dinners, pizzas, and other frozen products at the supermarket. It worked very well until she got married. Her new husband liked to have at least one meal a week made with fresh fruits, vegetables, and meat, and they cooked it together. As Adeline got better at cooking, she began to make more meals from fresh food products. Over time, her overall health improved, and she noticed that she was sleeping better. By the time she told me this story, she was only making one meal a week from processed food.

Not Getting Enough Variety

Eating the same foods at every meal is very easy but is not nutritionally sound. The nutrients that foods provide are unique to each food product. According to an article published by the Sleep Foundation in 2020, you will be better nourished if you include all the healthy foods you like in your diet on a regular basis. Eating the same meals every day can cause deficiencies in many of the micronutrients that your body needs for daily functioning, which impairs sleep. Processed foods also interfere with sleep. When you go to the supermarket, substitute some of the processed foods you'd normally buy with a couple of different vegetables and fruits each week. Eat different meats at each meal. Challenge yourself and try something new! You will sleep better when you get a variety of healthy, fresh foods that provide a variety of micro- and macronutrients.

Kyle went to the doctor for a routine checkup. His bloodwork revealed a low iron level. He was placed on iron with vitamin C. Three months later, his iron level was still low. His doctor sent him to a dietician who found that he had changed to a vegetarian diet. Previously he had eaten many red meats that supplied his body with iron. Kyle was counseled on how to change his diet, using vegetables to increase the iron in his bloodstream. He reported that he was sleeping better when his iron level rose. His doctor informed him that iron carries oxygen to the tissues, and because his tissues were better oxygenated, he was likely sleeping more calmly.

Tracking Your Progress

As you change your eating habits, use the attached habit tracker to help you to stay on course. You may try to keep a homemade copy in the kitchen so that while you are planning your meals, you are reminded what to avoid at certain times of the day. It will also remind you of some of the activities that will benefit you. Fill out your tracker daily to give yourself a record of your progress. Over time you will find that you do not want to lose your "streak" by skipping a day. The sense of well-being that comes from your progress is worthy of celebration.

HABIT	M	T	W	TH	F	SAT	S

KEY TAKEAWAYS

- Caffeine, alcohol, and carbohydrates can have an adverse effect on sleep.
- The body functions much more efficiently when you use fresh, healthy ingredients to fuel it.
- Choose low carbohydrate foods for lunch to help you maintain adequate wakefulness during the daily sleep dip.
- Timing meals appropriately affects sleep. The digestion process can interfere with sleep, so scheduling dinner four to five hours before bedtime to ensure digestion will help you to get to sleep and stay asleep much more easily.
- Food variety is important to obtain the necessary nutrients your body needs and to promote restful sleep.

CHAPTER 8

Taking a Technology Break

Technology is exciting. It provides information about what is happening in the world. It provides entertainment, escape, and distraction when we need it. It is a powerful communication tool that offers ways to stay in contact with friends and loved ones more easily than ever before. All good things have limitations, however, and electronics are no exception. Taking a break from these compelling devices is necessary for a calm mind and for healthy sleep.

Why Taking a Technology Break Matters

Electronic devices have changed our world in so many ways. Data about the world is now right at our fingertips and in our pockets. We no longer have to go to a physical place to find information, which frees up our time. The availability of information and connections with others allow for more sociability, as well.

Physiologically, electronic devices stimulate the brain with the blue light they produce (see chapters 4 and 5). They were made to keep us awake. They also elicit thoughts and responses to new data that keep the mind reeling. Responses to life events can be solicited from people from every possible perspective in a short amount of time. Information can be uploaded from any part of the world in real time. This onslaught of information can trigger emotions and even cause frenzied mental activity. For that reason, limiting the total time you spend on electronic devices is a good idea, and it's a particularly good idea to limit your time on devices prior to bedtime. A mind racing right before going to sleep results in difficulty getting to sleep, and the goal of improving your sleep habits is to calm brain activity in order to invite sleep.

The rule for this chapter is "no electronics one hour prior to bedtime." The equally important follow-up rule is "no electronics until you're out of bed in the morning." Simply avoiding electronics when you're preparing for bed and while you're in your bed will help you avoid the stimulation from the blue light and from information or entertainment that overstimulates your brain and your emotions when you should be sleeping.

Building Healthier Habits

The gradual yet continually accelerating nature of technological change means that many of us use technology for a rapidly increasing number of purposes, such as a tool for work, an entertainment and information source, and a way to communicate with others. Although many of the uses of technology are positive, it's also easy to suddenly find yourself using it all day long for work and nearly all evening for entertainment (while sometimes still occasionally checking email). Building intentional habits related to technology use can diffuse feelings of stress and urgency and restore a sense of balance and calm, both of which will increase the quality of your sleep. Healthy technology habits can also help you make time for other activities that have positive effects on sleep like getting regular exercise (chapter 6), meal planning (chapter 7), getting outdoors (chapter 10), and practicing mindfulness (chapter 11), not to mention other calming pursuits like writing, reading, or doing puzzles.

This set of habits helps you create appropriate associations between your brain and your bed. When you are able to get technology away from the area where you sleep, it's easier to resist the temptation to look at it, your sleep is not disrupted by notifications, and the bed becomes a place with a specific purpose. Developing good technology habits allows you to get the uninterrupted sleep you need for your mind and body to rest and reset for the day to come.

Schedule Device Time

This habit is creating intentional time limits for your use of your electronic devices. If you only allow yourself to use your devices within a specific time range, you will likely become more efficient in your work, and you will avoid exposure to light and a racing mind prior to bedtime or when you wake in the night. Over time, when you wake to use devices, your body learns to wake continuously at that time, which makes it much harder to stop the habit and maintain sleep.

Gina had been waking at 3:00 a.m. every night for the last six months. Initially she simply laid in bed and tried to get back to sleep. Over time, she began to pick up her cell phone and text friends, read her email, and play games. When she came to me, she was very sleepy because she had difficulty returning to sleep. She began to set an alarm on her cell phone for 90 minutes prior to bedtime. When the alarm sounded, she turned off her cell phone and the computer. She turned them on when she woke in the morning, after she had gotten out of bed. The break from technology in the evening and absence of technology in the bed area helped her to sleep much more soundly.

Set an alarm for 60 to 90 minutes prior to bedtime. Turn off all electronics, including electronic reading pads, computers, and cell phones. Begin your pre-bedtime routine. Your reward is getting to sleep easily and staying asleep well.

Turn the Television Off

Many individuals watch television in bed or leave the TV on all night. Television, similar to electronics, activates our mind. The TV interferes with getting to sleep and staying asleep because the volume of commercials is higher than programming. This has the potential to wake us or to bump us out of the deeper stages of sleep. Experts in sleep at Harvard Medical School report that the main problem with blue light is that it resets your circadian rhythm. Any exposure to light, simply by opening your eyes to roll over, or adjust bedding, have the potential to wake you and frequently shifts you into a lighter sleep for the remainder of the night.

Bob kept his TV on all night. He had done this since he was a teenager and had never noticed a problem with his sleep. He arrived in my office at age 45 and was very tired. After treating his sleep apnea, his sleepiness improved but was not within a normal range. He agreed to a trial of keeping his TV off at night for two months (he never had the volume turned up). When he returned, he was surprised and pleased to inform me that his sleep had dramatically improved.

Ideally, turn the television off one hour prior to bedtime when you turn off your other electronics. If you require background noise to fall asleep, white noise machines provide soothing sounds that can help. If you need light, standard night-lights will work. Your reward is getting good-quality sleep and feeling refreshed in the morning.

Enforce a "Do Not Disturb" Time

Allowing phone communication at any time of the day and night is not conducive to good sleep. If someone calls you in the middle of the night, disrupting your sleep and causing emotions to rise, your sleep quality suffers. It is a good idea to let your family, friends, and coworkers know when you are available for phone communication. Then, about an hour before bedtime, turn off your phone or put it on "do not disturb" and leave it on that setting until you get out of bed in the morning to ensure that you are not disturbed during the night.

Carol loved her job. The only thing she did not love about it was that she was on call every night of the week. When she received calls, they were often time-consuming and emotional, which caused her to have a very difficult time getting to sleep again. The calls were not necessarily emergencies—she simply needed to make decisions about next steps for first shift workers. She decided to inform her staff that she would not be available for calls after midnight or before 5:00 a.m. She turned off her phone during that period. She is sleeping much better now.

Inform family and friends and coworkers when you will take calls. Set a phone alarm for the time you turn off your phone. Set another alarm for the time you turn it on. Your reward is having a disturbance-free block of time for sleep.

Use a Conventional Alarm

Setting a conventional alarm to wake in the morning may seem inconvenient compared to using your phone alarm, but it is more conducive to sleep. If you have difficulty waking to an alarm, placing the alarm on the other side of the room is helpful. Some individuals need to gradually wake in the morning. In that instance, it is better to set several alarms than to continue to hit the snooze button, because the snooze tells the brain that it's okay to procrastinate.

Brenda was a night owl. She always had difficulty getting out of bed in the morning. She set 12 alarms on her phone to go off in five-minute increments. Sometimes she lost count of the alarms, did not get out of bed on time, and was late for work. She was told she would lose her job if she was late one more time. Her therapist suggested that she set one alarm (not on her phone) and put it across the room from her bed. She got out of bed when the alarm sounded and did not return. She was able to accept that first reminder to wake in the morning.

Get a conventional alarm. Turn it away from the bed so you cannot see what time it is in the night. Set it for the earliest time you need to get out of bed on any given day. When the alarm sounds, turn it off and get up. Your reward is an uninterrupted night's sleep.

Allow Only SIS in Bed

This final habit is the greatest reinforcement of creating a strong association for sleep with your bed. Follow the rule that the bed is only for sleep, intimacy, and sickness (SIS). If you wake in the night, the first thing you can try to do is basically clear your mind and bore yourself to sleep again. If you become uncomfortable lying awake, take the mental activity that you are experiencing out of the bedroom because the bed is only for SIS. Go to another room, and under dim light, do something that you know will put you to sleep. The activity must be calming and preferably boring. For example, read something boring. Then go to bed when you are sleepy. Avoid all technology during this time.

Jane often awakened in the night. She would lie in bed and try to get to sleep. When she was unsuccessful, she got up and watched TV until she got sleepy. Some nights she never returned to bed because she became so engaged in the TV show. When she came to see me, I suggested that she sit down and read the dictionary under a dim light. She was getting back to sleep quickly in no time because she wasn't giving her mind anything to enjoy.

If you wake in the night, avoid turning on any electronics and, instead, have a boring activity prepared ahead of time that you know will put you to sleep. Quietly do what you know has helped you get to sleep in the past and try to sleep again once you feel sleepy.

Breaking Bad Habits

Electronics are compelling. For most people, the attachment to technology and electronic devices is so strong that it becomes hard to turn them off. Because devices are intended to be stimulating and entertaining, they do not encourage relaxation or facilitate sleep. To sleep well, you must carve out time in your day when you do not have access to electronics, preferably before bed.

The most common technology bad habits include the following: playing games, texting or emailing on cell phones while in bed, keeping the TV on all night, using laptop computers in bed, using a cell phone as an alarm, and watching TV programs or movies on phones or tablets while in bed.

Light has a powerful effect on your circadian rhythm. In fact, many sleep clinicians use light to help individuals develop a normal sleep schedule. This is why light appears so frequently in these habits. I cannot emphasize enough that light exposure stimulates the brain and can wake you or keep you from getting into the deeper stages of sleep in an acceptable amount of time.

Creating Negative Associations with Your Bed

It is easy to become attached to the bed and want to spend more time there, especially when you're not sleeping well. Spending time in bed hoping sleep comes is detrimental. It allows the mind to make negative associations with the bed. Generally, this takes the form of using technology, fretting, worrying, and tossing and turning. To break this habit, substitute meditation or relaxation techniques for frustration and worry. These are positive, calming ways to distract and entertain yourself while you wait for sleep. Concentrating on your breath and counting backward from 100 is helpful. Listening to calming guided imagery or white noise can also invite sleep.

When I was in college living in dorms, I got into the habit of studying and writing papers on my laptop in bed. When I moved to an apartment and had space to move into another room, I felt more comfortable in bed doing my schoolwork. It worked well until I started having difficulty getting to sleep at night. I changed my habits after reading about sleep hygiene. Then I did my school-work at my desk and began to meditate for 15 minutes while lying in bed. Within 10 days, I was again getting to sleep easily; however, I had to be very strict with my schedule for several months.

Using the Cell Phone as an Alarm

One of the habits I see most frequently in my work is using the cell phone as an alarm. When the cell phone is used as an alarm, it is very conveniently located at the bedside for easy access. This means that if you wake in the night, it is very easy to give in to the temptation to look at your phone.

To get around this, you can use a conventional alarm, as mentioned earlier. In addition to that, it is very helpful to place your phone in another room, on the other end of the house, or on the other side of the bedroom. This ensures that you'll be less likely to get out of bed to use your phone in the night.

When April's daughter was in the ICU after a car accident, April got into the habit of having her phone nearby in the event the hospital would call and need something from her. If she woke in the night, she would check her phone to make sure she hadn't missed a call. As her daughter became healthier and moved out of the ICU and eventually returned home to recover, April found that when she woke in the night, it had become a habit to check her phone. She began to leave her phone in the kitchen when she went to bed at night and soon began sleeping through the night.

Tracking Your Progress

Monitoring your use of technology will help you become more efficient with it during the day. It will also help you sleep at night. Electronics are very difficult to resist, but avoiding their use during the time that you have blocked for relaxation and sleep will enhance your sleep quality and your ability to effectively unwind from your day. Keep track of your progress on the tracker to help some of these habits become automatic behaviors. Your reward will be better-quality sleep and well-functioning days.

HABIT	M	T	W	TH	F	SAT	S

KEY TAKEAWAYS

- Technology is a compelling tool. Not only does it enhance daily activities, but it also provides entertainment at all times of the day. Therefore, it has a powerful ability to negatively affect sleep habits.
- Setting boundaries for your use of technology and what is acceptable in your bed can help you get better quality sleep. This happens because you are limiting light exposure and avoiding anything but sleep, intimacy, and sickness in bed. This strengthens your mental associations between your bed and sleep.
- If you turn off your device one hour prior to bedtime and avoid turning it on again until you get out of bed in the morning, you reduce the temptation to use it if you awaken in the night. Sometimes placing your devices far away from your bed is necessary to help you avoid using them in the night.

CHAPTER 9

Managing Stress

We hear about stress management from all corners of society. Much of stress is how we think about the situation in which we find ourselves. The stress management habits in this chapter are designed to reshape how we think about stress. There is one stress management tool to which we will devote an entire chapter: mindfulness. We will discuss that topic in chapter 11.

Why Managing Stress Matters

There is a bidirectional relationship between stress and sleep. Experts are unsure which comes first, and it's likely unique to each individual. Sometimes sleep is poor because of stress. Sometimes poor sleep heightens anxiety and worry.

When episodic stress occurs, the brain releases hormones that largely consist of adrenaline and cortisol. These are the same hormones that enter the bloodstream during times of anxiety and panic as well as intense fear. Chronic stress is when a consistent stream of these stress hormones flow through the bloodstream. Chronic stress is associated with long-term stressful situations such as chronic illness, poverty, or abuse.

The constant presence of these hormones can cause damage to the body and mind. The body is at higher risk of developing high blood pressure, heart disease, cancer, and immune system deficiencies, and the mind is at risk of developing anxiety, depression, mood disorders, short-term memory loss, and the inability to focus.

Reduction of stress will help with your ability to sleep. Once stressors have been alleviated, sleep is more effortless. If your brain has been trained to react to stress, you can also train it to decompress. With habitual practice, stressors can be relieved or at least lessened by the habits in this chapter.

Retraining the brain is similar to other forms of training, like training your muscles to respond in a particular way. If you want to increase the size of your biceps, you can start a weightlifting program to do that. Retraining your brain is similar. The following habits retrain the brain to calm itself in spite of the problems that are present. When stressors arrive, all you need to do is remember your cue, and then you can invite a stress reducer into the situation.

Building Healthier Habits

Stress can be inhibiting, especially if it's bottled up and allowed to compound on itself. The key is to adopt healthy habits that help you release stress. Imagine that your body is a jar with the lid screwed on tight. Trapped in the jar are little molecules of stress, whizzing around with tremendous energy, crashing into the sides of the jar in an increasing frenzy. What happens when you open the lid? The molecules are released, and the inside of the jar becomes quiet and calm. The habits in this chapter are a way of opening the lid.

There are different approaches to releasing stress. Exercise, as you learned in chapter 6, is a great approach, and journaling, as I mentioned in chapter 3, is a great way to process your day, record your personal growth, and release stress before bedtime. Habits that help you see the world in a more positive way are also helpful, whether that means making sure to include some lighthearted fun in your day, retraining your brain to avoid getting worked up over small mistakes, or recognizing the good in the world by accepting help from others and offering help in return. In addition, you can develop habits of relaxation, meditation, or stretching that help you release the physical and mental tension you're experiencing.

It's likely you'll need to identify and develop a combination of habits. Your new habits can be spaced through the day, used as needed, or scheduled and stacked with other habits. You'll find that by creating habits that release stress, not only will you sleep better, but you will also enjoy an elevated mood, increased ability to focus, decreased illness and body pain, and even improved relationships.

Write in a Journal

To initiate this habit, ask yourself what specifically is causing your stress. It may be hard to answer but writing in detail about a specific experience or contingency is helpful so you can examine it later. It works best if you can write by hand in a paper journal. When you pair a mental exercise (composing) with a physical exercise (writing), your mind and body learn to work together, and stressors can be released in both places simultaneously.

Janet was an RN. She was stressed because of work (they were short-staffed) and Janet was picking up some duties that were easy for her but were also time-consuming. After a month, with no prospect of hiring additional help, she began to have difficulty sleeping and felt fatigued. She started writing in her journal. After a couple of weeks, reviewing her journal entries, she learned that she could reduce her stress by tweaking her process at work. She is still working hard and doing extra but is sleeping better and feeling a sense of accomplishment for figuring out her issue on her own.

Begin a journal, handwritten if possible. Your cue is a feeling of anxiety, fatigue, or headache accompanied by restlessness, feeling overwhelmed, a lack of motivation, mood swings, or difficulty sleeping. Your routine is to write a detailed journal entry. You may need to continue this routine daily for a week or two to begin feeling some release. Your reward is a calm mind and body that allow you to achieve better quality sleep.

Express Gratitude

When we can find things in our lives for which to be grateful, our emotions are automatically lifted. To develop this habit, begin by thinking about a negative situation and consider the benefits of the experience. For instance, the pandemic is a negative; however, we are learning how important social contact is and embracing new and creative ways to keep it present in our lives.

Jean studied very hard for her anatomy midterm, focusing on all the areas where she had previously done poorly. After the test, she thought that she had nearly aced it. She was devastated to find out that she got a 53 percent on her test. She did not sleep well that night. She made an appointment to review her responses with her professor, and they discovered that Jean had indeed gotten 96 percent of the questions correct. Failing the test was a negative, but Jean believed in herself enough to investigate, which turned out positively for her. This put her mind at ease and she was able to return to normal sleep.

Create a gratitude journal. This is a good habit to stack into your bedtime routine. Every evening, write about what you are grateful for and why. You could be grateful for your progress on beginning an exercise program for instance. One entry from my own journal states: "I am grateful for my worry because it reminds me what is important to me." Your life will become much more positive when you can be grateful for little things, even negative things.

Seek Out Laughter

Laughter truly does make the world a better place. Finding something to laugh about always lifts the mood and lightens the atmosphere. The act of laughing reduces stress by reducing blood pressure, anxiety, and depression, and it produces an overall sense of well-being. When you feel better about yourself, you can manage stressors with more grace and dignity. As a bonus, the reduction in anxiety and depression will help you sleep well at night.

When Vicky's mother became ill, Vicky took care of her. Vicky's mother initially became very upset when Vicky, who was not good at caring for another person full time, would laugh about her mistakes. When Vicky realized her mother was taking offense to her laughter, she talked with her, explaining that she laughed because she knew that she was making mistakes. As Vicky became better at what she was doing, the laughter died down. So, her mother started finding things to laugh about because she felt so much better when she was laughing. The stress of those early days caused many sleepless nights, but now that they are laughing together, they are also both sleeping much better.

Set aside time every day to look for things to laugh about. If you have difficulty finding humor, find a book of jokes or comedy shows on television to watch. Bring levity into your life—you will sleep better.

Practice Progressive Relaxation

Progressive relaxation is a form of relaxation in which you progressively move up or down your body flexing and relaxing muscle groups. This practice reduces stress by teaching your muscles how to relax. At first, it requires conscious effort, but over time it becomes automatic. First, relax in a sitting or lying position. Then, take deep cleansing breaths from the diaphragm. You should be able to see or feel your abdomen rising with each inhalation and falling with each exhalation. With every large muscle group, tense the muscles with a long inhalation and relax them with exhalation. If you start with the head, for example, scrunch up your facial muscles and relax them. Gradually work down the body: next flex the neck, then the shoulders, the arms, abdomen, buttocks, quadriceps and hamstrings, calf muscles, and feet. You'll notice as you relax these muscles that tension is released, which allows for more comfortable sleep.

Andrea noticed that her neck and shoulders were always sore when she was under stress and began to think about her posture. She realized she was holding herself as though she was constantly shrugging. When she woke at night feeling tension, she performed progressive muscle relaxation. She found that she was sleeping much better and feeling more rested when she was able to perform this ritual.

Sore or tense muscles at bedtime is your cue. Your routine is to perform progressive muscle relaxation as described above. Your reward is restful, tension-free sleep.

Practice Meditation

Meditation can be done in many ways and is widely known to relax the mind. If listening to your breath is easy for you, you may need no other props to perform meditation. If you do better with a supportive prop, there are many apps available and many meditation guides can be found online. Regardless of how you go about meditation, this tool has the capacity to calm the mind and establish peaceful feelings that invite sleep. Meditation exercises specifically for sleep can especially be helpful. Meditation works by resetting thought processes, making it easier to reframe your thoughts in a more positive way. By decluttering the mind and reducing racing thoughts, sleep becomes much easier.

Emily recently started a new job. She was learning so much at this new position that she found her mind racing at bedtime. She talked to her sister about the issue, and she suggested that she try meditation prior to bedtime to see if her mind would calm. Emily began practicing a meditation specifically for sleep that she found online. After a few days, she found it much easier to go to sleep and felt that she was getting deeper, more satisfying sleep.

Find a meditation resource that you think will work for you. At bedtime, begin your routine by listening to your meditation app or performing a breathing meditation. Over several days of persistent practice, you will get to sleep quickly and easily.

Breaking Bad Habits

It's common to try to alleviate stress by taking on additional activities, thinking that socializing or getting involved in a class or a group activity will help. Initially, it probably does help, but over time, an overbooked schedule will become another source of stress. This can be true in your personal life or in your work life. Overcommitment can appear to be a good coping strategy, but overcommitment is actually a way of not allowing enough time for ourselves.

On the other end of the spectrum, many people isolate themselves when they are under a great deal of stress. This is a form of self-protection. As social beings, this can be detrimental because it causes lost connections with others. Friends and loved ones, sometimes without your knowledge, help you carry your stress load just by knowing what you're going through. Though isolation provides you with more time, it is detrimental because you are not taking advantage of the natural support that others provide in your relationships. Accepting support from others is necessary for growth and change.

Overcommitment

Overcommitment is more common among extroverts. It is difficult to stop, especially if you are involved in group activities because of an obligation to people with whom you interact. There are ways to reduce your time commitment to a specific activity. However, sometimes regardless of how much you change this aspect of the activity, you remain stressed. An exercise to help you determine the benefits and shortcomings of your activities is to list all their benefits and obligations.

Next, prioritize the activities according to those that benefit you most and those that benefit you least. When you complete this exercise, you can decide which activities to stop or reduce your engagement in. When you reduce your time in an activity or stop engaging in the activity, you will have more time for self-care. As you reduce your activity level, stress levels will also go down and sleep will improve.

Ella is the mother of three girls. They are all in Girl Scouts. They are also engaged in several other activities, including dance, sports, and playdates. Ella was involved in the planning and organization of all of these things. Ella started to have difficulty sleeping at night. When she came to me, I suggested she prioritize the activities her girls participated in according to how she benefited from them. She ended up continuing to organize one activity for each daughter, only attending the other functions in which her daughters were involved, when necessary. Her stress levels took a precipitous dip, and Ella began sleeping better.

Isolation

Isolation is more common among introverts. This coping mechanism is harmful because depression and anxiety can be exacerbated by a lack of input from others. You see yourself best when you are interacting with other individuals because they mirror who you are. Without that mirror to see how you are doing each day, you risk turning further into yourself and isolating yourself more.

It is difficult for someone who enjoys being alone to invite others into their lives, but it is necessary for good mental health. To combat isolation, make a point to reach out to others. Family and friends are often helpful when they are aware of how you are feeling. Getting a pet is also a good idea, because pets tend to draw us out. Joining a club or a group that interests you is another positive option.

Jessica was an introvert and preferred her own company. This worked out well for her until she became stressed about work. She was asked to expand her job responsibilities. Though she had no difficulty doing the job, she felt overworked and stressed. She began to have difficulty getting to sleep and staying asleep because of racing thoughts about work that plagued her. Her family recognized that she was isolating herself and drew her out. When her father got her a puppy for her birthday, she substituted her worry about work with the joy of having a new companion. She began to sleep better and feel better.

Tracking Your Progress

Tracking your progress managing stress is very important, especially when you are feeling isolated. The habits in this chapter can provide new ways to deal with stress and invite sleep. Identify those that most appeal to you or that are most applicable to your life. Use the blank space at the bottom of the tracker to add any other good or bad habits you want to work on. The habit tracker will help you as you make stress management a habit.

HABIT	M	T	W	TH	F	SAT	S

KEY TAKEAWAYS

- Three ways to form habits that will help with sleep-interrupting stress are: writing a detailed description of the stressor on paper so you can go back to it to measure your growth and adjust your perceptions, reframing a situation in a positive way, and relaxing the body and mind to help facilitate getting to sleep and staying asleep.
- Gratitude and laughter help you reframe your thinking and bring levity to your life. The more you laugh and express gratitude, the less your sleep is interrupted by worry and regret.
- Meditation calms the mind. Progressive muscle relaxation calms the body. Both can help you get to sleep at night and can be repeated during periods of wakefulness in the middle of the night.

CHAPTER 10

Getting Outdoors

Spending time outside helps the body tune in to nature, and–you may be surprised to learn–it also can help you get to sleep at night. It seems that exposure to natural light has a significant effect on our bodies and our sleep rhythms. Though it is unclear how and why this is, a small 2013 study published in *Current Biology* verified that our circadian clock, the internal clock that governs our bodily processes throughout the day, tends to reset itself when we spend time outside.

Why Getting Outdoors Matters

Exposure to light has a powerful effect on the body. Artificial light and the light of nature are different because the light of the sun is complex, and the light's quality changes over the course of the day. Morning light is thought to be blue-green, which has a more profound effect on our circadian clock. Blue-green light gradually decreases during the day, and there is some evidence that this blue-green morning light affects us differently than afternoon light. The red-orange light of the afternoon has less effect on our circadian clocks, likely because the body is already beginning its slow descent into relaxation and sleep. As red-orange light increases in the natural world, the time for the release of melatonin shortens.

A great deal of the artificial light you're exposed to during the day is blue light. With artificial blue light, you are exposed to the same quality of light all day. This stimulates the brain and suppresses melatonin production, which reduces the ability to get to sleep. Blue light gets turned off and on, providing no opportunity for the body to adjust its secretion of melatonin. The circadian rhythm misalignment caused by artificial light results in circadian rhythm sleep disorders. Therefore, reducing your exposure to artificial light and increasing your exposure to natural light improves sleep.

In the 2013 study referenced earlier in this chapter, participants spent a week in nature without artificial light and smartphones. Without them, they found that their body clocks had reset to be in rhythm with nature. In other words, exposure to blue-green light in the morning, the gradual change to red-orange light in the afternoon, and the natural darkness allowed their bodies to reset to nature's clock. A later study, conducted by some of the same researchers and published in *Current Biology* in 2017, tested participants after only a weekend in natural light and found that circadian realignment with nature occurred after only a few days.

Building Healthier Habits

Sometimes the motivation to get outside can be challenging if you haven't developed the habit, especially if you feel pressure to spend your workday indoors at your desk. But making time to get outside before or after work, or even for a short break will make a difference at the end of the day when it is time to go to sleep. Generally, morning light is thought to be more beneficial than afternoon light. Therefore, getting outside in the morning will be most helpful; however, getting outside more at any time of day is beneficial.

Many of us have a renewed appreciation for the outdoors after experiencing various stages of lockdown due to the COVID-19 pandemic. You may have discovered that you enjoy eating outdoors, even if you have to bundle up a little bit in cooler weather. Or you may have discovered that hiking or picnicking in a park, instead of a movie marathon, is the way you love to spend your Saturdays. Or you may find that sitting on the front steps and chatting with neighbors helps ground you during stressful times.

Regardless of the specific habits you develop, as long as you're getting outdoors, you will experience myriad benefits for your life—and your sleep.

The habits in this chapter will start your creative juices flowing when it comes to finding ways to get outside each day. You may choose to adopt some or all of these habits or to think up some on your own. The important parts of this process are spending the time and effort to develop the habit, tracking your progress to ensure success, and enjoying the time you spend outdoors.

Take a Walk

Walking is a great excuse to get outside. You can walk to the shops or the market, through a park, to a friend's house, on the golf course, or along the beach. Or mix it up! There are so many possibilities. You don't have to walk fast or walk for a long time. The point is to get outdoors. Getting into the habit of walking is also fairly simple as I explained in the gradually increasing duration habit (page 71) in chapter 6. For those who are unable to walk, getting outside in a wheelchair (or with other types of assistance) or simply sitting on the porch, is also a great option.

Sandy walked every day on her treadmill. She started using her treadmill in the winter when it was cold and just kept walking indoors through the summer. One day a friend asked her to go for a walk with her. Sandy enjoyed the walk outside, noting how things had changed in the neighborhood since she had stopped walking outdoors. That night, she had no difficulty getting to sleep. She started walking outside every day that the weather was good and now sleeps much better as a result.

Choose the best time of day for you to take a walk. The time of day will be your cue. At some point, tying your walking shoes or putting on your walking clothes may be your cue. Go for a five-minute walk. Every day add one minute to your walk. In one month, you will be walking 30 minutes. Your reward is getting to sleep quickly and waking feeling more refreshed.

Park at the End of the Lot

We all need to shop for things—groceries, hardware, home supplies, and so on. When we park in the lot of our favorite stores, we often try to find the closest parking spot. Instead, look for the parking spot farthest away from the entrance of the store. This gives you some exercise time outside. If you plan shopping trips in the morning, you will also get the benefit of the blue-green light, which will help you wake up and stay alert for the remainder of the day.

Harry needed to get time in the sun because his vitamin D level was low, but he had little time to spend outside. He was a regional manager of a store chain and spent many of his days going from store to store to deal with problems. He started parking at the far end of the parking lot. He figured that this habit alone gave him about 35 extra minutes outside. His vitamin D level increased, and he started sleeping much better, as well.

Your cue is a trip to the store. Park at the far end of the parking lot and walk the extra distance to the entrance. This is your routine. Your reward is getting better sleep because you spent more time outside.

Read Outdoors

Many people enjoy reading or looking at magazines in the house with a favorite drink and their feet propped on an ottoman. But think how easily this time could be spent outside on a nice day, either on a porch or sitting on a park bench. If you have a covered area, you could do this even on a rainy day. Begin by spending five minutes outside with your favorite reading material or puzzle book. Add one minute each day and you will soon be spending 30 minutes outdoors.

Brayden loved to read. He spent hours on his couch reading his favorite books and magazines. He was told by his physician that he needed to spend more time outside because he began having difficulty getting to sleep at night. A close look at his sleep hygiene had revealed that there was no other issue that needed adjustment. Brayden began to spend 30 to 60 minutes of his time reading outside. Within a few days, he was getting to sleep much more quickly.

Choose a time of day that you typically pick up a book, magazine, or puzzle book. The time of day will be your cue. Substitute time spent reading indoors with time spent reading outside. Begin with five minutes. Add one minute each day. This is your routine. Your reward is improved sleep.

Eat Outdoors

An easy way to spend time outside is to eat a meal or two outdoors every week. When making meal plans for the week, you might eat takeout at a picnic table or on the porch. This provides for time outside and will also help reset your circadian clock on a regular basis. You can also barbecue outside if you are so inclined.

Amelia regularly barbecued two to three times per week in the spring, summer, and fall months. She noticed that she did not sleep as well in the cold winter months. She came to see me because she wanted a sleeping medication for the winter months. As we explored her sleep schedule and habits related to sleep, the only thing that changed was that she stopped spending as much time outside in the winter because of the cold weather. She began to cook outside again at noon two to three days per week, spending as much time outside as she could comfortably, and found that she began to once again sleep much better.

Plan to eat two or three meals per week outside. Your cue is your meal plan. Your routine is eating outside. Your reward is ease at getting to sleep and staying asleep.

Explore Your World

Plan one or two days per week to spend some time exploring something outside that you are interested in learning more about. There are many activities that can be done outside that satisfy your curiosity and expand your world. Some of these include bird watching, looking at flowers or other plant life, finding out what lives under a rock, looking for four-leaf clovers in the lawn, and observing how the seasons change.

Jill quit one of her jobs so that she could spend more time at home with her children. She and her two boys all had some difficulty with getting to sleep at night. Jill began to plan outdoor scavenger hunts with her children. They spent two to three hours per day outside when she planned these events. She noticed that her children were getting to sleep much better when they spent time outside. Now, though they do not have a scavenger hunt every day, they spend a substantial amount of time outside.

Think about something outside that you would like to learn more about. Schedule a time one day a week to explore your interest. When you are doing this routinely once a week, add a new interest and spend two days a week exploring. This activity ties in nicely with mindfulness, which we will discuss in further detail in chapter 11.

Breaking Bad Habits

There are many compelling reasons to avoid going outside and most have to do with comfort. Indoors, we can control the lighting, temperature, sounds, and smells in our surroundings. That is much more unrealistic when we are outside. With technology that makes our indoor lives so much more comfortable, going outside is no longer as soothing as it once was. If you really wish to improve your health and your sleep, however, you will need to do some things that are outside of your comfort zone. Spending time outdoors may be one of those things.

Part of the discomfort with the outdoors may stem from failing to have the right equipment. Appropriate footwear, clothing, and other supplies can keep us comfortable outside. You may need to have several different outfits for your outdoor escapades to align with the changing seasons. Lack of preparation makes the activity less enjoyable and makes you less likely to return to that activity later.

Being Unprepared

Being unprepared for an activity is one of the most common problems with outdoor activities. Doing activities outside may require you to invest in some simple equipment. For instance, a water bottle to stay hydrated, activity-appropriate footwear, and healthy snacks if you plan to be out for a long time. Being prepared for adverse weather and for minor injuries is also important. Sunscreen and bug spray may be needed supplies. Being prepared by having these basic, inexpensive supplies at the ready will make your outdoor activity much more enjoyable.

Adam loved to hike. He recalled when he first started going on hikes that he forgot something each time he went out. To rectify this, Adam began making lists of what he took when he went hiking. He soon had a master list that he, to this day, checks every time he goes hiking. He is much more comfortable, and his hikes are much more enjoyable now. He has always recognized an association between his outdoor activities and his ability to sleep well. He sees it as one of the perks of staying active.

Lacking Motivation

It is easy to resist spending time outside, as so much immediate gratification often lies in the comfort of our homes. To break this habit and build your motivation, you will do what you have done frequently with previous habits—build on your successes. Begin by simply spending a short period of time outside. Each day, add a minute of time to your routine. In this way, you'll gradually increase your time outside. If you can add an enjoyable activity to this time outside, you will be more likely to continue the practice.

Ellen loved watching birds. When the weather was too hot or cold, she stayed indoors to watch them through her windows. When the weather improved, she found it so much more comfortable to stay inside watching birds. She started noticing that her increased time indoors had a negative effect on her sleep and her digestive rhythms. She once again began watching birds outside and found that within just a few days she was feeling better and sleeping better.

Tracking Your Progress

As you track your progress with getting outdoors, note the time of day and the duration of time you spent outside. By recording these two data points, you can keep closer track of your progress. You might also consider tracking your sleep to see what time of day being outside most benefits you and how the duration of time you spent outside affects the quality of your sleep.

HABIT	M	T	W	TH	F	SAT	S

KEY TAKEAWAYS

- Spending time outside resets your circadian clock and improves many of your bodily rhythms. In addition, it can help ward off disease and improve your sleep.
- Overexposure to artificial light, particularly blue light, has many negative effects on the body. Exposure to artificial light also has been implicated in circadian rhythm disorders. Getting exposure to natural light can help you avoid these effects.
- Adding time outdoors to your normal schedule is a convenient way to increase your time outside. Partaking in enjoyable activities outside can reduce the time it takes to get to sleep and help you stay asleep at night.

CHAPTER 11

Practicing Mindfulness

Mindfulness is the practice of purposeful awareness. This can take the form of meditation, relaxation, or an intentional focus on your surroundings. Mindfulness is thought to strengthen your ability to relax and is a good practice when you are preparing for or maintaining sleep. Mindfulness techniques have the ability to enhance all daily activities, especially when it helps you relax.

Why Practicing Mindfulness Matters

Mindfulness techniques were initially developed in Buddhist and Tibetan meditation practices. In the 1970s, these techniques were further developed for use in clinical psychology and psychiatry by academics at the Stress Reduction Clinic at the University of Massachusetts. They have used mindfulness to treat depression, stress, anxiety, and drug addiction. Mindfulness has since been studied and found to have profound benefits on mental health.

As you learned in chapter 9, when you reduce stress and anxiety, your sleep will naturally improve. Mindfulness helps reduce negative thinking or ruminations about worrisome or anxiety-producing issues. Because these tendencies often occur prior to bedtime or when we wake in the night, mindfulness is an especially powerful sleep tool.

The Mayo Clinic encourages practicing mindfulness for 20 minutes a day. This duration has been known to increase attention span, improve sleep, stabilize blood sugars, and reduce the tendency to be judgmental. It has also been effective at reducing stress, anxiety, depression, insomnia, and pain. Everyone has the capacity to be mindful.

Practicing daily will make these benefits more available to you. When it is easy to access the mindful state, it will be easier and more automatic for the mind to relax into sleep at bedtime or upon waking in the night.

Mindfulness, because it is focused on the here and now, also promotes acceptance and a lack of judgment about what is happening around us. You can develop a healthy curiosity about the world through mindfulness because you are looking at the world as it is in the current moment and accepting it as it is. You also will more readily observe the subtle changes around you, which can teach you more about yourself and your environment. The acceptance and suspension of judgment allows the mind to relax more easily. When the mind relaxes more easily, it is much easier to get to sleep.

Building Healthier Habits

Mindfulness can be practiced in a couple of different ways. One way is to focus on the breath during meditation, which encourages relaxation by raising your awareness of your body. Another way to practice mindfulness is to sit quietly and pay attention to your thoughts, without judgment or analysis. Simply watch your thoughts float by, acknowledge them, and let them go. This method of treating your thoughts with acceptance allows you to keep emotions at bay so you can relax and simply be.

You will be able to better develop some of the mindfulness habits in this chapter, especially if the concept and practice are new to you, if you do them in a specific time and place every time. Other habits, however, can be used on the go. Just remember, as with other new habits, it is important to start simply, work up gradually, and set achievable goals.

After you review the habits in this chapter, you may find that they are beneficial in many different scenarios, including for relaxation during your bedtime routine, for falling asleep once you're in bed, for getting back to sleep after waking in the night, and even for starting your day in the morning. You may find that one habit works best for relaxation, while a different habit may be particularly effective at soothing a specific emotion when it arises. The process of finding what works best for you in a given situation may take a little trial and error, but the powerful benefits of mindfulness on your sleep—and on your life—are worth the effort.

Focus on the Breath

Focusing on your breathing and regulating your breathing can help you relax and stay in the moment. Notice how your muscles move and how the air feels rushing through your nose. Notice how your chest feels when your lungs are full compared to how it feels when your lungs are deflated. Your mind should be focused solely on your breath and breathing. You should feel your body relax as you breathe in and out. As your body begins to relax, so will your mind.

Raphael had two jobs and had to be in bed within an hour after getting home from his second job so he would be able to wake up in time to get to his first job. His work schedule was difficult, but even more difficult was getting to sleep at night after a busy day. His brother had a similar problem and started focusing on his breath before bedtime, and the practice was very successful for helping him get to sleep. Raphael tried it and found that it worked beautifully for him, too. He now is having no difficulty getting to sleep, even after a busy and hectic day.

Your bedtime routine or getting into bed at bedtime is your cue. Your routine is to take a few minutes to focus on your breath. Feel your body relax. Continue this for as long as you are comfortable. Your reward is getting to sleep with ease.

Observe Your Thoughts

Paying attention to your thoughts and releasing them, without analysis or judgment, causes relaxation. Making predictions about what may occur next in life using personal experience and knowledge as a guide is a natural human response. Some predictions are based on fears and concerns about the future or the past. When you can release these fear-based thoughts, you will find it much easier to relax. This can be especially important in the later parts of the day when it's common to feel fatigued or to feel that your defenses are down. The more often you can practice the habit of releasing negativity and expectations when you are feeling strong, the easier it will be to perform the habit when you are stressed.

Jacob complained that his mind raced at night. He noted that the thoughts he had in the evening were more negative than his daytime thoughts. He decided to try a unique form of guided imagery in which he placed every negative thought on a helium balloon and let it float away into the clouds. The more practiced he became with the technique, the easier he was able to rid his mind of negative thinking prior to sleep, which made getting to sleep much easier for him.

During your bedtime routine, take a few minutes to focus on your thoughts. Pay attention to them, but do not dwell on them. Allow them to pass freely in and out of your mind. Feel free to use the guided imagery that Jacob used if it helps you release your thoughts. Feel your mind relax. Your reward is a relaxed mind that is prepared for sleep.

Live in the Moment

In our busy lives, it is easy to overlook what is occurring around us when we are bombarded with stimuli. But if you take some time to absorb the sights, sounds, smells, and tactile sensations in your immediate environment, your anxieties can dissipate. The more practice you get, the more automatic the habit will become, which allows you to slow yourself down and access a sense of calm when you need it most.

Chelsea came to see me because she was having difficulty getting to sleep at night. Her bedtime routine was not helping her. When we delved into why, we learned that she was being distracted by thoughts of past negative experiences. She would worry about her responses to questions at work and become anxious about how she had been seen by others. She began to practice living in the moment and discovered that when she was focused on her task, her brain did not distract her. Now she has no difficulty remaining focused on her bedtime routine.

Begin by looking around you and focusing on what you see, recognizing objects and their qualities. What do you smell? Is there any noise where you are in this moment? Touch objects and feel the warmth and the texture of their surface. How does your body feel in this moment? Are you enveloped by a sense of calm? Do this several times a day and your reward will be the ability slip into living in the moment much easier in the future.

Do a Body Scan

A body scan can be done while sitting or while performing an activity like walking. Regardless of how you choose to perform this task, you will be consciously scanning every muscle group, every organ, every system in the body for what you feel in those areas. If you do this while walking, you might focus on the timing and sensation of flexion and relaxation of muscle groups. If you are sitting, you might take note of how your muscles feel on the hard or soft surface you are perched upon.

Hank was looking for a mindfulness technique he could perform in his wheelchair. He liked the idea of checking in with his body because even though he was a hemiplegic, he still had phantom pains and aches and wanted to see if focusing in on those areas would reduce the pain he felt. He started doing body scans every day. Within a few weeks, he noticed that his phantom pain issues were reduced, and he was also sleeping better.

If you are walking, choose a short 10- to 20-foot route that you can walk very slowly, paying attention to your muscle groups and how they are functioning. If you are sitting, you will pay attention to your muscle groups at rest. The reward for this habit is feeling relaxed and in the moment, which will keep your mind at ease when you are ready to fall asleep.

Observe the Environment for Changes

This habit can be done when you are actively doing something else like walking, running, biking, hiking, or driving. It is especially helpful when you are on a route that you take often. As you proceed down the road or path, observe (to the extent that it's safe for you and those around you) the environment for any changes that have occurred since you last visited the area. Often birds or wildlife will draw attention. Sometimes a yard or home has changed in some way, or flowers in the yard have bloomed. Note how your mind and body feel as you are focusing on these changes.

My family lives in Iowa, and I live in Tennessee. Two to three times a year, I drive to Iowa to visit my family. On the trip, I often practice mindfulness by observing changes in cityscapes and landscapes. Each season brings out different types of wildlife and bird life. Instead of this being a boring or tiring trip, it often energizes me. I also always find that the first night in Iowa is a great night for sleep.

When you are doing something that takes you along the same route repeatedly, observe the environment for changes that have occurred since you were last in the area. Use all your senses. Pay attention to how your body feels when you are focused on your environment. This intense focus of the mind is rewarded at bedtime when you fall right to sleep and sleep soundly through the night.

Breaking Bad Habits

Paying attention to what you are doing and what is going on around you are good things most of the time. Mindfulness includes two simultaneous actions: paying attention to your surroundings and practicing acceptance while withholding judgment. However, if you don't engage with both parts of this equation, you can slip into some bad habits. Being nonjudgmental about your thoughts and what is occurring around you is a difficult task, especially in a world so fraught with criticism and a lack of empathy.

Even though an aspect of effective meditation is practicing acceptance and not making judgments, you are *capable* of making judgments while meditating. It is important to try to resist this.

You can also become less motivated or less willing to take responsibility for your actions when meditating. Acceptance without a willingness to act on your knowledge is not a good thing. A 2019 study published in the *European Journal of Social Psychology* examined whether moral decision-making is affected by mindfulness. The authors found that mindfulness decreases the desire to restore a situation to its previously normal state. In other words, mindfulness can make you less likely to fix problems and more likely to accept them as they are. It is important to understand this and to consider how you can avoid being oblivious to the need to behave responsibly.

Remaining Judgmental

Paying attention to your surroundings but remaining judgmental is not true mindfulness, yet often happens when you begin a new practice. Being nonjudgmental is so important because it allows the brain to relax rather than maintaining a tense state of assessment. It can be difficult to relax enough to allow simple acceptance, but it is necessary to obtain the softening of mental processes you need for quality relaxation and sleep.

Releasing judgment has a soothing effect on the brain and the body. Paying attention to your body when you are tense about an issue will make you better able to recognize when you are passing judgment rather than allowing acceptance. Reducing judgment reduces stress, and stress reduction leads to better sleep.

Charlotte was experiencing insomnia because she was having difficulty releasing her feelings of being hurt by her best friend. She decided to start a gratitude journal in which she tried to find something good in every situation—even difficult situations. She found that as she wrote, she was able to see the good in the pain she was feeling and recognized that she was part of the problem because she was being judgmental about the argument with her friend. When she realized this, she was suddenly able to sleep better once again.

Avoiding Responsibility

Acceptance of the state we find ourselves in is thought to be a good trait. However, when we accept behaviors that are harmful, especially over the long term, we are doing ourselves and others damage.

Over the long term, acceptance of negativity can reduce your quality of life. You also may find it difficult to raise yourself out of your situation. Acceptance needs to be coupled with an effort to repair the damages done in the situation. It is possible to accept your circumstances and still ameliorate the harms that come with a particular event.

Hilary was living in the moment. She felt calmer and freer when she could allow circumstances to play out naturally. When her son was bullied by a classmate, she accepted what was going on and was present for him as he talked about the situation with her. Over time, her son began to act out at home and Hilary began to lose sleep over the situation. She talked her position over with a counselor who encouraged her to stand up for her son, emphasizing that acceptance did not mean that you do not act. Her son is now doing well, and Hilary is sleeping well again.

Tracking Your Progress

Like the previous activities discussed in this book, mindfulness is best learned through repetition until it becomes an automatic behavior. If you have already had some success with the previous habit trackers, this one will be equally helpful. You may not engage in all of these activities, but tracking the ones you do perform will help you to make them automatic.

HABIT	M	T	W	TH	F	SAT	S

KEY TAKEAWAYS

- Mindfulness is a powerful tool to treat various conditions such as depression, stress, anxiety, and drug addiction, because it calms the brain and thereby initiates relaxation and sleep.
- Mindfulness can take many different forms and can be done in many different ways and circumstances. It is always a conscious effort to take in your surroundings and the state of your body.
- There are two parts to mindfulness: focusing on the here and now and accepting the circumstances in which you find yourself. Acceptance doesn't mean that you do not act. It means that you do not judge.
- Mindfulness relaxes the mind by releasing negative thoughts and ruminations and focusing on the present moment. Mindfulness reduces the feeling of being drained by your worries and your fears.
- Being mindful for a short period of time every day trains your brain to relax at will. Being mindful prior to bedtime trains your brain to relax into sleep.

RESOURCES

Books

Alexandre, Renata. *The Sleep Workbook: Easy Strategies to Break the Anxiety-Insomnia Cycle*. Emeryville, CA: Rockridge Press, 2020.

Clear, James. *Atomic Habits: An Easy and Proven Way to Build Good Habits and Break Bad Ones*. London: Penguin Random House, 2018.

Duhigg, Charles. *The Power of Habit: Why We Do What We Do in Life and Business*. New York: Random House, 2012.

Epstein, Lawrence. *A Good Night's Sleep*. New York: McGraw-Hill, 2007.

Martin, Paul. *Counting Sheep: The Science and Pleasures of Sleep and Dreams*. New York: Thomas Dunne Books, 2002.

Walker, Matthew. *Why We Sleep: Unlocking the Power of Sleep and Dreams*. New York: Scribner, 2017.

Apps

Mindfulness Coach: An app developed for veterans by the U.S. Veteran's Administration

Buddhify: An app that contains guided meditations

Guided Mind: An app that contains guided meditations

Calm: An app that helps users improve sleep quality

White Noise Deep Sleep Sounds: A white noise app

Insight Timer: An app for sleep, meditation, and relaxation

REFERENCES

Alexandre, Renata. *The Sleep Workbook: Easy Strategies to Break the Anxiety-Insomnia Cycle*. Emeryville, CA: Rockridge Press, 2020.

American Stroke Association. "Sleep." American Heart Association. March 19, 2019. www.stroke.org/en/about-stroke/effects-of-stroke /physical-effects-of-stroke/physical-impact/sleep.

Barrett, Lisa Feldman. *How Emotions Are Made: The Secret Life of the Brain*. Boston: Mariner Books, 2018.

Carpenter, Michael. "How Outdoor Activities Affect Our Sleep." rtor.org. June 1, 2020. www.rtor.org/2020/06/01/how-do-outdoor-activities -affect-our-sleep.

Chellappa, Sarah L., Roland Steiner, Peter Oelhafen, Dieter Lang, Thomas Götz, Julia Krebs, and Christian Cajochen. "Acute Exposure to Evening Blue-Enriched Light Impacts on Human Sleep." *Journal of Sleep Research* 5, no. 22 (October 2013): 573–80. doi:10.1111/jsr.12050.

Cho, YongMin, Seung-Hun Ryu, Byeo Ri Lee, Kyung Hee Kim, Eunil Lee, and Jaewook Choi. "Effects of Artificial Light at Night on Human Health: A Literature Review of Observational and Experimental Studies Applied to Exposure Assessment." *Chronobiology International* 9, no. 32 (September 2015): 1294–310. doi:10.3109/07420528 .2015.1073158.

Clear, James. *Atomic Habits: An Easy and Proven Way to Build Good Habits and Break Bad Ones*. London: Penguin Random House, 2018.

Cleveland Clinic. "Insomnia." Last updated October 15, 2020. my .clevelandclinic.org/health/diseases/12119-insomnia.

Duhigg, Charles. *The Power of Habit: Why We Do What We Do in Life and Business*. New York: Random House, 2012.

Epstein, Lawrence. *A Good Night's Sleep*. New York: McGraw-Hill, 2007.

Goodheart, Annette. *Laughter Therapy: How to Laugh About Everything in Your Life That Isn't Really Funny*. Santa Barbara, CA: Less Stress Press, 1994.

Hafenbrack, Andrew C., and Kathleen D. Vohs. "Mindfulness Meditation Impairs Task Motivation but Not Performance." *Organizational Behavior and Human Decision Processes* 147 (July 2018): 1–15. doi:10.1016/j.obhdp.2018.05.001.

Harvard Medical School. "External Factors that Influence Sleep." *Healthy Sleep*. December 18, 2007. healthysleep.med.harvard.edu/healthy/science/how/external-factors.

Heid, Markham. "How Do the Bacteria in My Gut Affect My Sleep?" *Everyday Health*. Last updated February 24, 2020. www.everydayhealth.com/sleep/how-do-the-bacteria-in-my-gut-affect-my-sleep.

Khalsa, Sat Bir S., Stephanie M. Shorter, Stephen Cope, Grace Wyshak, and Elyse Sklar. "Yoga Ameliorates Performance Anxiety and Mood Disturbance in Young Professional Musicians." *Applied Psychophysiology Biofeedback* 34, no. 4 (December 2009): 279–89. doi:10.1007/s10484-009-9103-4.

King, Brian. *The Habits of Stress-Resilient People*. Seminar presented in Nashville, TN, on October 15, 2019.

King, Brian. *The Laughing Cure*. New York: Skyhorse Publishing, 2016.

Langille, Jesse J. "Remembering to Forget: A Dual Role for Sleep Oscillations in Memory Consolidation and Forgetting." *Cellular Neuroscience* 13, no. 71. (March 12, 2019). doi:10.3389/fncel.2019.00071.

Martin, Paul. *Counting Sheep: The Science and Pleasures of Sleep and Dreams*. New York: Thomas Dunne Books, 2002.

Mateo, Ashley. "The Intimate Relationship Between Fitness and Sleep." *Everyday Health*. May 23, 2018. www.everydayhealth.com/fitness /intimate-relationship-between-fitness-sleep/.

Murray, Kate, Suneeta Godbole, Loki Natarajan, Kelsie Full, J. Aaron Hipp, Karen Glanz, Jonathan Mitchell, Francine Laden, Peter James, Mirja Quante, et al. "The Relations Between Sleep, Time of Physical Activity, and Time Outdoors Among Adult Women." *PLoS One* 9, no. 12 (2017): e0182013. doi:10.1371/journal.pone.0182013.

National Traffic Highway Safety Administration. "Drowsy Driving." United States Department of Transportation. www.nhtsa.gov/risky-driving /drowsy-driving.

Norton, Amy. "Time Outdoors May Deliver Better Sleep." *Web MD*. February 2, 2017. www.webmd.com/sleep-disorders/news /20170202/time-outdoors-may-deliver-better-sleep.

Pacheco, Danielle. "Exercise and Sleep." *Sleep Foundation*. Updated January 22, 2021. www.sleepfoundation.org/physical-activity /exercise-and-sleep.

Rasch, Bjorn, and Jan Born. "About Sleep's Role in Memory." *Physiology Review* 93, no. 2, (April 1, 2013), 681–766. doi:10.1152/physrev .00032.2012.

Schindler, Simon, Stefan Pfattheicher, and Marc-André Reinhard. "Potential Negative Consequences of Mindfulness in the Moral Domain." *European Journal of Social Psychology* 5, no. 49 (January 2019): 1055–69. doi:10.1002/ejsp.2570.

Shechter, Ari, Elijah Wookhyun Kim, Marie-Pierre St-Onge, and Andrew J. Westwood. "Blocking Nocturnal Blue Light for Insomnia: A Randomized Controlled Trial." *Journal of Psychiatric Research*, 96 (2018): 196–202. doi:10.1016/j.jpsychires.2017.10.015.

Smith, Lori. "What Are Binaural Beats, and How Do They Work?" *Medical News Today*. September 30, 2019. www.medicalnewstoday.com /articles/320019.

Sparks, Dana. "Mayo Mindfulness: How Mindfulness Helps You Live in the Moment." *Mayo Clinic: News Network*. April 25, 2018. newsnetwork .mayoclinic.org/discussion/mayo-mindfulness-how-mindfulness -helps-you-live-in-the-moment.

Stothard, Ellen R., Andrew W. McHill, Christopher M. Depner, Brian R. Birks, Thomas M. Moehlman, Hannah K. Ritchie, Jacob R. Guzzetti, Evan D. Chinoy, Monique K. LeBourgeois, John Axelsson, and Kenneth P. Wright Jr. "Circadian Entrainment to the Natural Light-Dark Cycle across Seasons and the Weekend." *Current Biology* 27, no. 4 (February 2017): 508–13. doi: 10.1016/j.cub.2016.12.041.

Suni, Eric. "Nutrition and Sleep." *Sleep Foundation*. Updated November 6, 2020. www.sleepfoundation.org/nutrition.

Walker, Matthew. *Why We Sleep: Unlocking the Power of Sleep and Dreams*. New York: Scribner, 2017.

Wein, Harrison, ed. "Sleep On It." *NIH News in Health Newsletter*. April 2013. newsinhealth.nih.gov/2013/04/sleep-it.

Wright, Kenneth P., Jr., Andrew W. McHill, Brian R. Birks, Brandon R. Griffin, Thomas Rusterholz, and Evan D. Chinoy. "Entrainment of the Human Circadian Clock to the Natural Light-Dark Cycle." *Current Biology* 23, no. 16 (August 2013): 1554–58. doi: 10.1016/j.cub.2013.06.039.

INDEX

Acknowledgments

I would like to thank all my friends and colleagues at St. Thomas Sleep Specialists for their patience and forbearance as I worked on this book. They helped me out in so many ways to keep my workplace efficient while I was writing. I would also like to thank my neighbors for their help while I wrote this book. I also appreciate the help of my editor, who has been supportive and very helpful with her comments. And last, but not least, I would like to thank all the patients who have expressed support for my writing endeavors. I thank you all from the bottom of my heart.

About the Author

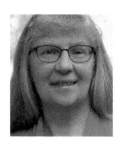

Renata Alexandre is a certified nurse practitioner who holds a PhD in health and human performance and has master's degrees in nursing, divinity, and sociology. Clinically her passion is sleep medicine. She has specialized training in cognitive behavioral therapy for insomnia and has been practicing for 13 years. She is the author of *The Sleep Workbook: Easy Strategies to Break the Anxiety-Insomnia Cycle*. When she is not working or writing, she likes to garden, hike, read, and listen to music. She lives in Nashville, Tennessee.